MW00606736

PROGRESS IN CLINICAL RHEUMATOLOGY

VOLUME 1

PROGRESS IN CLINICAL RHEUMATOLOGY

VOLUME 1

Edited by

ALAN S. COHEN, M.D.
Conrad Wesselhoeft Professor of Medicine, Boston University School of Medicine; Chief of Medicine and Director, Thorndike Memorial Laboratory, Boston City Hospital, Boston, Massachusetts

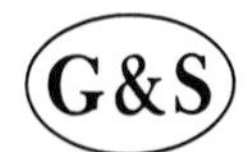

GRUNE & STRATTON INC.
(Harcourt Brace Jovanovich, Publishers)
Orlando San Diego San Francisco New York London
Toronto Montreal Sydney Tokyo São Paulo

Grune & Stratton, Inc.
Orlando, FL 32887

Distributed in the United Kingdom by
Grune & Stratton, Ltd.
24/28 Oval Road, London NW 1

International Standard Serial Number 0742-745X
International Standard Book Number 0-8089-1646-7
Printed in the United States of America
84 85 86 87 10 9 8 7 6 5 4 3 2 1

Contents

Preface

The rheumatologic literature has expanded enormously in the past 20 years. There exist a multiplicity of medical journals both in the United States and abroad, and many original articles in the field are published in general research or clinically oriented journals as well. *Progress in Clinical Rheumatology* is designed to provide timely and comprehensive reviews of major clinical topics; of investigative topics relevant to our understanding of the clinical state of the art; and to bring to bear our understanding of basic considerations on the clinical and therapeutic aspects of the particular disorder.

In this first volume, each of the above has been attempted. Chapter 1 presents an in depth review, based on animal models and basic modern immunologic science, of the conceptualization of systemic lupus erythematosus. Dr. Steinberg, a major contributor to our understanding of this increasingly complex area, gives the reader a clear understanding of current concepts of host factors, immune factors, and genetic factors as primary or secondary phenomena in SLE.

In Chapter 2, Drs. Nepom and Schaller analyze in detail their extensive personal experience with childhood SLE. They review not only the clinical manifestations, but laboratory studies, modes of treatment and prognosis, as well as neonatal lupus.

Chapter 3 combines the physiologic and therapeutic approaches. Drs. Kahaleh and LeRoy review not only the natural history and clinical manifestations of the disease, but stress the basic factors that may be related to its pathogenesis. The vascular disorder in scleroderma is lucidly discussed as well as the fibrotic, collagen related aspects and immunologic phenomena that occur.

In recent years aggressive treatment for rheumatoid arthritis has been increasingly emphasized. Drs. Klinenberg, Reichman, and Clements appropriately entitle this "Investigational Therapy" and expound in a precise fashion the current status of the use of azathioprine, 6 mercaptopurine, cyclophosphamide, chlorambucil, methotrexate, thoracic duct drainage, apheresis (plasmapheresis, cryopheresis, etc), and total lymphoid irradiation. They provide us with information about the mechanism of action, toxicity, and therapeutic results that will be a springboard for the understanding of future studies.

Another disease in which technology has made a major impact albeit in diagnosis rather than therapy, is ankylosing spondylitis. Drs. Khan and Kushner after a useful clinical review evaluate the current approach to the diagnosis of spondylitis. Radiographs, computerized tomography, radionuclide scintigraphy, thermography, nuclear magnetic resonance, and finally the role of HLA-B27 testing are discussed. The use of sensitivity-specificity testing allows a clearer appreciation of the value of the HLA-B27 test.

Finally, Drs. Goldenberg and Rice review one of the most treatable forms of articular disease, acute gonococcal arthritis. They update what had been controversial regarding the sequential clinical stages of the disease and discuss diagnosis and treatment. Of particular note is their review of the new data on the microbial and host features of disseminated gonococcal disease and the role of immune mechanisms, and then discussion of a new laboratory model. It is through studies such as these, that we shall obtain a better understanding of the epidemiology of this worldwide disorder.

Thus the reviews in Volume I of *Progress in Clinical Rheumatology* deal with problems in the major connective tissue diseases, i.e. rheumatoid arthritis, systemic lupus erythematosus, scleroderma, ankylosing spondylitis, and infectious arthritis.

Alan S. Cohen, M.D.

Contributors

ALAN S. COHEN, M.D., *Conrad Wesselhoeft Professor of Medicine, Boston University School of Medicine; Chief of Medicine and Director, Thorndike Memorial Laboratory, Boston City Hospital, Boston, Massachusetts*

PHILLIP J. CLEMENTS, M.D., *Assistant Adjunct Professor of Medicine, UCLA School of Medicine; Division of Rheumatology, Cedars-Sinai Medical Center, Los Angeles, California*

DON L. GOLDENBERG, M.D., *Associate Professor of Medicine, Boston University School of Medicine; Associate Director, Medical Service, Boston City Hospital, Boston, Massachusetts*

M. B. KAHALEH, M.D., *Associate Professor of Medicine, Department of Rheumatology and Immunology, Medical University of South Carolina, Charleston, South Carolina*

MUHAMMAD A. KHAN, M.D., *Associate Professor of Medicine, Case Western Reserve University; Division of Rheumatology, Cleveland Metropolitan General Hospital, Cleveland, Ohio*

JAMES R. KLINENBERG, M.D., *Professor of Medicine, UCLA School of Medicine; Director, Department of Medicine, Cedars-Sinai Medical Center, Los Angeles, California*

IRVING KUSHNER, M.D., *Professor of Medicine, Case Western Reserve University; Division of Rheumatology, Cleveland Metropolitan General Hospital, Cleveland, Ohio*

E. CARWILE LEROY, M.D., *Professor of Medicine, Director, Division of Rheumatology and Immunology, Medical Center of South Carolina, Charleston, South Carolina*

BARBARA S. NEPOM, M.D., *Fellow in Pediatric Rheumatology, Department of Pediatrics, Division of Rheumatology, Children's Orthopedic Hospital, Seattle, Washington*

RONALD REICHMAN, M.D., *Assistant Clinical Professor of Medicine, UCLA School of Medicine; Division of Rheumatology, Cedars-Sinai Medical Center, Los Angeles, California*

PETER A. RICE, M.D., *Associate Professor of Medicine, Boston University School of Medicine; Infectious Disease Section, Boston City Hospital, Boston, Massachusetts*

JANE G. SCHALLER, M.D., *Professor and Chairman, Department of Pediatrics, Tufts-New England Medical Center, Boston, Massachusetts*

ALFRED D. STEINBERG, M.D., *Chief of Cellular Immunology Section, Arthritis and Rheumatism Branch, National Institute of Health, Bethesda, Maryland*

PROGRESS IN CLINICAL RHEUMATOLOGY

VOLUME 1

Alfred D. Steinberg

1
Modern Concepts of Systemic Lupus Erythematosus

Systemic lupus erythematosus (SLE) is a spontaneously occurring non-specific disorder of the organs that has a tremendous variability of expression. People of all ages may be affected; however, females between the ages of 12 and 40 are most often afflicted. In addition to the spontaneous occurrence of SLE, the disease may be induced in humans by administration of certain drugs. Not only humans develop SLE; but also many other mammals, including dogs, mink, and mice, develop the syndrome. We will try herein to describe the current conceptual framework for the development of autoimmune diseases in general and systemic lupus in particular. Next, we will describe the information available from studies of animals with SLE as a background for discussing the human disorder. Human SLE will be described in terms of immune regulatory abnormalities, organ pathology, current approaches to treatment, and potential newer modalities.

THE CONCEPTUAL FRAMEWORK FOR THE DEVELOPMENT OF AUTOIMMUNE DISEASES

How does an autoimmune disease occur? Does each have the same general basis? Do all patients with SLE have the same regulatory defect or the same pathogenetic mechanisms? These questions cannot be answered definitively at present. Nevertheless, a substantial increase in the knowledge of immunology and molecular biology allows us to consider the general problem of autoimmune disorders.

PROGRESS IN CLINICAL RHEUMATOLOGY VOL. I ISBN 0-8089-1646-7

Until recently, it was thought that anti-self reactions were abnormal and detrimental. More recently, however, it has become apparent that self-self recognition plays an important role in normal immune responsiveness and homeostasis. Cells of the immune system recognize specific major histocompatibility complex (MHC) encoded recognition structures during the process of responding to specific foreign antigens. Antibodies to foreign antigens (Ab_1) give rise to antibodies specific for themselves (Ab_2). Such anti-idiotype antibodies have the capacity to regulate immune responses to the antigen to which Ab_1 reacts. Ab_2 can recognize cells with receptors that bear the idiotype of Ab_1 as well as recognizing secreted Ab_1. Therefore, there is a great range of possible regulatory interactions in this system. In addition, antibody itself (Ab_1) is capable of exerting feedback regulation. Both antibodies and cells, thus, can recognize self-determinants and play a role in normal regulatory processes.

How does this new knowledge affect our concepts of autoimmune diseases? It makes us realize that autoimmunity is common, normal, and not pathological (Table 1-1). Only when autoimmune reactions lead to tissue damage or some other pathological disorder is the process abnormal and disease inducing. In other words, autoimmunity is not at all abnormal. It is part of the normal regulatory activity of the immune system. As a result, autoimmune reactions and autoimmune phenomena are not, in themselves, pathological. This recognition makes us distinguish between noninjurious and injurious autoimmune phenomena. As a corollary, there may be autoimmune phenomena that do not serve any normal regulatory processes but that are not injurious. For example, many healthy people have antibodies reactive with nuclear antigens, immunoglobulins, thyroid antigens, etc. but do not suffer obvious ill effects of such antibodies. These people may be viewed as manifesting abnormal autoimmune phenomena without manifesting illness. The recognition of nonpathogenic autoantibodies allows us to appreciate that patients with SLE may have many deleterious autoantibodies but that some of their autoantibodies may not be pathogenic. Thus, from the viewpoint of understanding pathogenesis, special emphasis must go to those antibodies that induce injury and/or inflammation. Similarly, those are the antibodies against which therapy must be directed. The same holds for nonantibody-mediated inflammatory processes.

THE MULTIFACTORIAL NATURE OF DISEASE INDUCTION

Common sense and numerous observations point to multiple factors in the development of many diseases. It is clear that miliary tuberculosis (TB) is "caused" by the tubercle bacillus. It is also clear that Ashkenase Jews rarely develop miliary TB and that on exposure to TB, Eskimos and Alaskan Indians often develop miliary TB. Therefore, other factors, in this case

Table 1-1
Concepts of Immune Regulation and Their Relationship to Autoimmunity and Autoimmune Diseases

1. Self–self interactions form the bases for both normal immune reactions and normal immune regulation.
2. These self–self interactions include self-recognition by parts of the immune activity on the basis of that recognition.
3. Since #2 represents an autoimmune response, autoimmune responses are part of normal physiology.
4. Diseases associated with autoimmune responses can result from a variety of different types of abnormalities
   a. A defect in the afferent limb of the immune system initiated without a requirement for a specific external agent
      With important genetic requirements
      Without important genetic requirements
   b. A defect in the afferent limb of the immune system initiated by a specific external agent
      With important genetic requirements
      Without important genetic requirements
   c. A defect in effector mechanisms of immunity initiated without a requirement for a specific external agent
   d. A defect in effector mechanisms of immunity initiated by a specific external agent
   e. Combinations of a–d
5. Many autoimmune diseases are multifactoral in etiology and/or disease expression.
   a. Genetic—Disease is often polygenic
      —Individual genes predispose to particular abnormalities
   b. Environmental factors—Stimulate the immune system (specifically or polyclonally)
      —Interfere with normal immune regulation
   c. Hormonal factors—Modify disease manifestations

apparently genetic factors, may predispose to, or protect against, the development of a disease. This is true whether or not there is a specific "etiologic" organism. Additional factors clearly predispose to miliary TB. These include, but are not limited to, degree of crowding, alcoholism, nutritional status, immunosuppressive events, immunostimulatory events, and prior exposure. In other words, miliary TB may be viewed as multifactorial in etiology, despite the necessary requirement for the tubercle bacillus. In fact, the genetic factors may be so important in some populations that it may be viewed as a genetic disorder as much as an infectious disorder. One could even do genetic analyses of populations and families and try to determine the genetic basis for susceptibility. The take-home message is that even for a disease with known "triggers," multiple factors may determine whether the disease will be manifested.

How does this apply to SLE? It appears that SLE is a disorder in which multiple factors combine to determine whether disease will be expressed and to what extent. In some individuals, the genetic predisposition may be so strong that trivial environmental factors or even no environmental factors may be necessary for the disease to be expressed. In other individuals, the genetic predisposition may be modest; moderately strong environmental factors may be required for disease expression. Additional factors, such as sex hormone metabolism and state of the immune system, may be sufficient to allow or prevent disease expression. Clues to the multifactorial nature of SLE in a given individual and to the differing factors in different individuals come from studies of mice that spontaneously develop SLE.

MURINE SYSTEMIC LUPUS

For physicians who are interested only in the management of human SLE, there is a strong tendency to skip over sections such as this. That is a most unfortunate tendency since more is known about murine SLE, and what is known can be applied to human lupus. Unlike other diseases in which there are animal models that provide little insight into the human disorder, murine SLE occurs spontaneously, has characteristics of humans with SLE, and responds to therapy the way patients do.[1] Most important, the ability to dissect the genetic basis for illness and the pathogenesis of immune abnormalities is much easier and more advanced in murine systemic lupus. One cannot, therefore, be a fully informed physician of patients with SLE without a working knowledge of the disease as it occurs in mice.

Mice with systemic lupus come in different sizes and colors. Their MHC types may be different.[1–4] In other words, the genetic basis for illness may be different in different mice with lupus (Table 1-2). The most commonly studied mice have been the New Zealand black (NZB), (NZB × NZW) F_1, MRL-*lpr*/*lpr*, and BXSB. These mice have differences in the pace of illness and sex hormone effects. The BXSB mice have a male-oriented illness; the males have accelerated disease relative to the females. Some factor associated with the Y chromosome of the BXSB mouse appears to be responsible. Sex hormones are not able to reverse this male disease.[5] However, whereas the BXSB Y chromosome leads to disease in BXSB mice and in male offspring of BXSB males with autoimmune-prone females, the BXSB Y chromosome does not lead to accelerated disease in offspring of BXSB fathers and non-autoimmune-prone mothers.[6] Therefore, the BXSB Y chromosome factor is an accelerating factor rather than a lupus-inducing factor.

Another accelerating factor is the *lpr* gene. Originally described on the MRL background, this gene has now been bred onto many backgrounds.[4] In homozygous form, this gene leads to lymphoproliferation. The proliferating cell is a dull Ly 1 + T cell (helper phenotype).[7] Eventually, massive lymph-

Table 1-2
Heterogeneity of Murine Lupus

Feature	NZB	(NZB × NZW)F_1	MRL-MP/*lpr*/*lpr*	BXSB
Genetic	At least 6 autosomal genes	Multiple genes, some from NZW	Multiple background genes, *lpr* major accelerator	Multiple background genes, y chromosome gene major accelerator
Major histocompatibility	d/d	d/z	k/k	b/b
Sex	Little effect Recessive gene for androgen insensitivity	Marked effect Androgens protect Estrogens worsen	Androgens protect slightly	Marked acceleration in males, not hormonal
Immunoglobulins	↑ IgM	↑ IgM, ↑ IgG_2	↑ IgG_1, ↑ IgG2a	↑ IgG_1, ↑ IgG2b
Lymphoid organs	Lymphoid hyperplasia	Lymphoid hyperplasia	Marked ↑ T cells	Moderate ↑ B cells
Effects of *xid*	Prevents disease	Prevents disease	Retards disease	Prevents disease
Disease manifestations	Anti-T cell antibodies Coombs-positive hemolytic anemia Late life renal disease Splenic hyperdiploidy Death occurs after 1 year	Anti-DNA, LE cells Membranoproliferative glomerulonephritis Sjögren's syndrome Females die in first year of life	Marked lymphadenopathy Anti-DNA, anti-Sm Arthritis and anti-Ig Membranoproliferative glomerulonephritis Vasculitis Males and females die in first year of life	Immune complex glomerulonephritis Degenerative coronary artery disease Serologically less abnormal than others Moderate adenopathy Males die in first year of life

adenopathy and splenomegaly result. Female sex hormones are an accelerating factor and androgens are a retarding factor in (NZB × NZW) F_1 mice.[8,9] Females have much more rapid onset of disease and death than their male counterparts; however, that difference can be reversed by opposite sex hormone treatment. NZB mice tend to have late onset "middle-age" lupus with only a small difference between males and females. Some of these features are summarized in Table 1-3.

Of considerable interest are mice about which little has been written. These (NZB × normal) F_1 mice develop autoantibodies but usually live a normal life span. The (NZB × MRL) F_1 mice develop a milder disease than either parent. This stands in contrast to the (NZB × NZW) F_1 female, which gets a more severe disease than either parent. Gene interactions, thus, may give rise to either accelerated or retarded disease in offspring. These results have particular importance for human family and population studies. In

Table 1-3
Genetics of Murine Autoimmunity: Relationship to Human SLE

	Murine system	Human SLE
NZB	Inherited autoimmune traits with a lack of sex differences[4]	Familial incidence of SLE[2] Concordance in identical twins[3]
F_1 hybrids with NZB	Androgens suppress and mask genetic mechanisms[4]	Female predominance in SLE[1,2]
BXSB	Male-linked inheritance[1,30,39]	Inheritance of male predominant SLE[7]
Recombinant inbreds, lines of NZB × Normal	Independent inheritance of many autoimmune traits[8]	Familial members of SLE patients develop some autoimmune features without clinical SLE
F_1 and backcross analysis	Dominant and recessive inheritance of autoimmune traits with additional modifying genes. Many genes show gene dosage effects	Dominant inheritance of ANA and Anti-ssDNA.[5] Two genes may give greater abnormality than one.
Modifying factors *xid* gene retards	Predisposing factors.[37,56,71,90] Retarding factors[32,34]	B-cell hyperactivity in SLE[36,94]

addition, in mice it is clear that high titers of autoantibodies may be associated with a normal life span without therapy.

A careful analysis of the genetic basis for disease in NZB mice by use of F_1 and backcross mice has indicated that genes for anti-DNA and anti-T-cell antibodies are unlinked and coded for by single dominant or codominant genes.[10] Additional genes from the NZW mouse contribute to disease in the (NZB × NZW) F_1.[11] More recently, studies of recombinant inbred lines of mice derived originally from NZB and normals have indicated that multiple genes are responsible for the full disease of NZB mice. At least six genes contribute to the disease of NZB mice.[12] A similar analysis of background genes in MRL and BXSB mice would be helpful.

In addition to those factors mentioned previously, congenital factors other than mammalian genes may be critical to the expression of disease. An oncornavirus may cause accelerated disease by virtue of increasing the load of pathogenic immune complexes.[13,14] Such a virus in an animal with a defect in tolerance, thus, could induce antiviral antibodies and exacerbate immune complex disease. Although such a virus is not necessary for disease,[15] it could be a factor similar to other viral infections.[16] Another factor is a maternally transmitted antigen, which is present in some, but not all, mice. This antigen may result from cytoplasmic genetic material, which is passed on from the mother's egg. Mice with the antigen may be protected from the full expression of autoimmune disease.

The detailed analysis of the cellular bases for illness in the different strains of mice that develop lupus is beyond the scope of this chapter. It is helpful, nevertheless, to point out some of the findings. First, the role of the thymus in retarding or preventing disease in the different strains may be very different. Neonatal thymectomy of MRL-*lpr*/*lpr* mice has a profoundly ameliorating effect on disease. These mice, which ordinarily die at about 6 months of age, are essentially cured by neonatal thymectomy.[17] In contrast, neonatal thymectomy causes accelerated disease in BXSB males.[18] In our hands, neonatal thymectomy has a less dramatic retarding effect in NZB mice and an accelerating effect in (NZB × NZW) F_1 mice. The mouse strains, thus, must differ in terms of the cellular basis for illness if neonatal thymectomy can have such dramatically different effects in the different strains. These differences are explainable. The proliferation observed in MRL-*lpr*/*lpr* mice is primarily one of T cells. These T cells cannot proliferate without a thymus; therefore, neonatal thymectomy prevents disease. A corollary is that the autoantibody production is T-cell dependent. In contrast, most of the proliferation of BXSB mice is of B cells. The thymus ordinarily holds the proliferation of these B cells in check, albeit not completely. Neonatal thymectomy allows the B cells to proliferate in an uninhibited fashion; this gives rise to massive lymphoproliferation and markedly increased autoantibody production.

Immune Abnormalities That Lead to Disease versus Those That Result from Disease

In the mice, it is relatively easy to study individuals prior to the onset of clinical illness and then after illness occurs. Such studies clearly indicate that there are many immune abnormalities. Those that are found at the time of clinical illness, however, may not be those that set off the process. This concept is especially important because patients with SLE are rarely studied prior to the onset of symptoms. Abnormalities observed at the time of active disease are given great importance with regard to pathogenesis of the disorder. Some of these may, in fact, serve to perpetuate the disease process. They may not have been important, however, in its initiation. Antigen nonspecific suppressor function thus falls prematurely early in the life of the (NZB × NZW) F_1 mouse but rises abnormally after the onset of disease.[19] It is possible that the abnormality observed at the time of illness—increased suppression—is important in perpetuating the process; however, it has nothing to do with its initiation. In fact, increased suppressor function probably results from the markedly increased immune reactivity that is observed as autoimmune disease develops. The marked hyperactivity is, however, not adequately controlled by the reactive suppressor factors.

What can be said of the early abnormalities of mice with murine lupus? It appears, in general, that all have a stem-cell disorder. That is, they have defects that may be expressed in mature cells of the immune system but that are encoded in the stem cells and that can be transferred with stem cells.[20–24] The precise defects may be different in the different mice. A defect associated with T-cell proliferation, thus, is associated with MRL-*lpr/lpr* stem cells.[25] Similarly, a defect for interference with normal tolerance is characteristic of NZB pre-T-cell stem cells.[26] In both cases, the stem cells must be acted on by a thymus for the defect to be expressed. In contrast, non-T cells appear to be critical to the failure of normal tolerance and disease expression in the BXSB male.[27] The defects in the mature lymphoid cells thus may differ even though the information for the defects may be present in the stem cells in all of the mice.

Many abnormalities are observed late in the course of disease. These include autoantibody production, immune complex renal disease, impaired responsiveness to T-cell mitogens, and impaired IL-2 production. Impaired immune responsiveness to exogenous stimulation is found in association with vigorous immune activity during the course of the autoimmune process. In other words, at the same time that there is vigorous B-cell activity and production of autoantibodies, immune responsiveness to stimulation with nonspecific mitogens or foreign antigens may be markedly impaired. This paradox may be viewed teleologically as follows: the body is preoccupied with making autoantibodies and autoimmune responses and cannot be bothered with the new stimuli. At a more mechanistic level, two explanations are available. First, the autoimmune process leads to the production of vigorous immunosuppressive signals, which impair the responses to foreign antigens and mitogens. Second (and not mutually exclusive), pre-B-cell stem-cell pool is preempted by the maturation into autoantibody-producing cells and the T cells are functionally inactivated by suppressor factors, many secreted by nonlymphoid mononuclear cells. Additional factors occur in some, but not all individuals: anti-T-cell antibodies interfere with T-cell regulation. These various defects may be partly overcome by treatment with immunosuppressive regimens (including cortiocosteroids and cyclophosphamide) to restore more normal immune function. The problem, therefore, is not just a deficiency of adequate numbers of particular lymphocytes but active interference with normal cellular function.

HUMAN SYSTEMIC LUPUS ERYTHEMATOSUS: APPROACH BASED ON THE MURINE STUDIES

In the next several sections, information regarding human SLE lymphocytes will be put forth. An attempt will be made throughout to place the data in the perspective derived from the murine studies. This perspective includes the idea that different individuals with SLE may have different genetic and cellular bases for illness, that immune abnormalities observed during the course of active disease may not be those that induced the disease, and that many immune abnormalities may actually result from the disease process. Finally, throughout it must be appreciated that most studies of humans have been limited to the sampling of peripheral blood, whereas those of animals involve lymphoid organs such as spleen and lymph nodes and sophisticated transfer studies between experimental animals.

Lymphoid Cells in Patients with Systemic Lupus Erythematosus

Patients with active SLE often have leukopenia.[28] Although this leukopenia is accounted for on an absolute basis primarily by a reduction in granulocytes, there is also an absolute reduction in lymphocytes. There is thus the paradox of an increased percentage of lymphocytes in the differential but a decreased absolute number of lymphocytes on the basis of lymphocytes for each cubic millimeter of peripheral blood. Individuals vary greatly. Some patients have a leukocytosis, even without steroid therapy. Others have profound leukopenia, which may actually improve with immunosuppressive drug therapy.

Peripheral blood lymphocyte counts may be greatly depressed, in the normal range, or increased. In active disease, the average lymphocyte count was reduced approximately 70 percent, with approximately equal reductions in B and T cells.[29] That led to relative increase in cells of the monocyte–

macrophage series. In other words, patients with SLE have a relative decrease in lymphocytes among their peripheral blood mononuclear cells (Table 1-4). If studies, therefore, are performed on peripheral blood mononuclear cells (without further cell separation), there will be a relatively stronger influence of the nonlymphoid cells. This is especially important since such cells may exert profound suppressive influences.[30,31] A variety of in vitro tests may record impaired immune function solely because of this relative increase in the monocytes–macrophage series.

B-Cell Functions in Systemic Lupus Erythematosus

Patients with active SLE are characterized by hypergammaglobulinemia[32–38] and the production of large amounts of various autoantibodies (see below). Such patients have circulating cells that resemble activated lymphocytes,[39–42] which are able to produce immunoglobulin (Ig) after removal from the blood.[43] Such antibody-forming cells have been studied by a reverse hemolytic plaque technique, which allows enumeration of Ig-secreting cells of different classes. These studies have demonstrated marked increase in Ig-secreting cells in patients with active SLE.[44–50] Of interest, IgG- and IgA-antibody forming cells were markedly increased, whereas IgM often were not.[44,45]. Moreover, the degree of increase in antibody secreting cells was highly correlated with disease activity.[45] Of interest, numbers of IgG-secreting cells correlated better with disease activity than did anti-DNA, C3, and other classical serological measures.[51] Moreover, the Ig-secreting cells correlated in that study with multisystem disease activity but not with major organ involvement. In other words, arthritis and serositis were as likely to be associated with large numbers of IgG-secreting cells as renal or central nervous system disease (the latter were only associated if the disease was recently reactivated).

It might be anticipated from previous mention that all of the Ig-secreting cells were secreting autoantibodies. Although this is possible, it has been found that patients with active SLE have Ig-secreting cells of many different specificities,[52–54] many being chemical haptens to which the patients might not have been expected to have been exposed.[53,54] These results suggest that the patients are polyclonally activated and that the antibodies are not all directed at autoantigens (Table 1-4). One caveat remains: it is possible that unexpected cross-reactivities between the chemical haptens are masking the true hyperproduction of only autoantibodies. Although we feel that this is not a likely explanation, recent studies on the cross-reactivity of monoclonal antibodies leaves open this possibility (see also below).[55–59]

We thus find that in active SLE, patients manifest large amounts of antibody production, much of which is autoantibody. The exact amount of autoantibody is difficult to quantitate in many patients. As much as 4 mg/ml anti-DNA has been found in the serum of a patient with active SLE.[60] As a

Table 1-4
Immune Abnormalities in Systemic Lupus Patients*

Immune measures	Active disease	Inactive disease
Lymphopenia	+ + + + ↓	+ ↓
Absolute numbers of T cells	+ + + + ↓	+ ↓
Absolute numbers of B cells	+ + + ↓	0
Percentage of T cells	+ + ↓	± ↓
Percentage of B cells	+ + ↑	+ ↑
Percentage of T_G cells	+ + + ↓	± ↓
Skin tests	+ + + + ↓	+ ↓
Responses to Con A (proliferation + others)	+ + + + ↓	+ + ↓
Responses to PHA	+ + + ↓	+ ↓
Responses to PWM	+ + + ↓	+ ↓
Suppressor function (T cell)	+ + + + ↓	+ ↓
Macrophage–monocyte suppression	+ + ↑	+ ↑
Helper T-cell function	+ + + + ↓	+ ↓
B-cell proliferation (spontaneous)	+ + + ↑	+ + ↑
B-cell differentiation (Ig production)	+ + + + ↑	+ ↑
Marrow proliferation	+ + + ↑	+ ↑
Natural killer cell activity	+ + + ↓	+ ↓

↑ = increase; ↓ = decrease; 0 = no change; + = small; + + = moderate; + + + = large; + + + + = very large. All comparisons are with normals.
*Since human SLE is very heterogeneous and patients differ markedly, these generalizations are those of the majority of patients; exceptions are found.

result, it is possible that some patients have enormous amounts of autoantibody, which could account for the majority of their excessive immunoglobulin production.

Despite the known hypergammaglobulinemia and increase in spontaneous antibody-forming cells, the greater the disease activity, the poorer the response of SLE mononuclear cells to stimulation with the B-cell mitogen pokeweed mitogen.[48,50,61] In fact, patients with active SLE frequently have impaired B-cell responses relative to normals. The basis for the impairment is complex; however, the phenomenon is only superficially paradoxical. It is clear that patients with active SLE have in vivo activation of cells. It is not really a great surprise that such cells cannot be activated in vitro. If many cells have already proliferated and differentiated in vivo, those would be unable to provide much of a contribution following in vitro stimulation. Moreover, macrophages can suppress the responses in SLE or in T-cell populations in vitro.

Some authors have emphasized the known requirement for helper T cells in the pokeweed response of B cells and the defective helper T-cell function of patients with SLE,[6,48] which will be discussed below. Stimulation with a T-cell independent B-cell mitogen showed a relatively normal response in a few patients.[48] It is possible, therefore, that multiple mechanisms may be responsible for the impaired B-cell responses in vitro. Drs. Grayson, Blaese, and I followed a few such patients with active SLE and impaired responsiveness to pokeweed. We found that in a given patient different mechanisms of impaired responsiveness predominated in this same patient at different times despite no change in either disease activity or treatment.

In vivo studies of patients' B-cell functions are, like many of the in vitro studies, affected by changes in other cell populations. This may be the explanation for lack of uniform results. Patients have had normal[62–64] or decreased[65] antibody titers, which follows immunization with influenza vaccine. The primary responses were much more blunted than were secondary responses. Similar results were obtained following immunization with brucella and with KLH antigens.[37,66] In these studies, IgG responses were normal, but IgM responses were subnormal. This is consistent with an impaired primary and normal secondary response; however, it could represent a defect specifically in IgM responses. Normal antibody responses, obtained after immunization with tetanus toxoid and rickettsiae, would be secondary responses.[67]

Normal[68] or elevated[69,70] antibody levels without specific immunization were found for blood group antigens and penicillin *Proteus* OX-2.[37] Decreased resting antibody titers were found for influenza,[65] *Escherichia coli,*[37] *Shigella,*[37] and streptolysin O.[68] A number of papers have emphasized the elevated titers of antibody reactive with a variety of viral antigens;[71–75] however, not all of these may be real, as some of the assays allow SLE autoantibodies to react with cellular materials in the viral antigen preparations so as to yield a false-positive test.[76] Moreover, since SLE patients have preferential decreases in IgM responses, any assay that is especially sensitive to IgM antibody (e.g., hemagglutination or hemolysis) might show a decreased titer due to the particular class of antibody produced.

The in vivo studies suggest that patients with active SLE have impaired primary and IgM antibody responses to immunization but that they have normal or even elevated secondary and IgG responses. A similar impairment of primary responses and normal secondary responses has been observed in the NZB mouse model of SLE[2,77] with regard to both antibody production and skin graft survival. It appears that for both mice and people two explanations are available. One is that the ongoing autoimmune response leads to production of nonspecific suppressor factors as in antigenic competition.[78] This phenomenon is mediated by suppressor cells and can be eliminated with low doses of cyclophosphamide. The second explanation involves the known defects in helper T-cell functions, functions that may be necessary to a much greater extent in primary as compared with secondary responses (e.g., growth factor production). Primary responses are, moreover, much more easily suppressed than are secondary responses. Multiple immunizations, therefore, may be necessary to achieve the desired antibody response.

Studies of B-cell proliferation as opposed to Ig secretion, have also provided important information with regard to the B-cell functions in SLE. Patients with active SLE often have B cells with impaired proliferative responses to pokeweed mitogen in vitro, a defect that may relate to impaired T-cell help. Much more interesting are studies of spontaneous proliferation, since such studies might provide a clue to the in vivo situation.

A much greater degree of spontaneous proliferation of SLE B-cell enriched fractions was observed when studied right out of the body than after 3 days in culture.[29,79] Of interest in that study, patients with inactive SLE demonstrated as much proliferation as did patients with active SLE. The difference, therefore, between inactive SLE and active SLE appears to be a signal that induces the B cells to start to differentiate into immunoglobulin-secreting cells. Such a signal, however, takes place in the context of already proliferating B cells. Activation, therefore, does not require a signal for proliferation, only one for differentiation. It is possible that SLE B cells are more susceptible to such a trigger by virtue of altered membrane potential or an increase in the number of receptors for T-cell factors.

Patients who go into prolonged remission may revert toward normal and then require signals for both proliferation and differentiation in order to develop B-cell hyperactivity.

Recent studies of stem cells in SLE suggest that the B-cell hyperactivity has a basis in increased stem-cell activity. Patients with SLE were found to have increased numbers of B-cell colony-forming cells.[80] This increase was independent of T-cell function; in fact, the ability of SLE T cells to support colonies was impaired. More recent studies by Dr. Laskin (unpublished data) have indicated that patients with active SLE have a fivefold increase in numbers of marrow stem cells at the end of 1 week in Dexter cultures in vitro.

T-Cell Functions in Systemic Lupus Erythematosus

A very large number of studies have evaluated T-cells and T-cell functions. The first question is whether the amazing B-cell hyperproliferation and hypersecretion can be related to abnormally active T-cell help. Many years ago we attempted to study this question in collaboration with Dr. T. Waldmann and found that patients with active SLE had markedly impaired help for polyclonal immunoglobulin production (unpublished). More recently, similar observations have been published.[6] It therefore appears that in the majority of patients, excess T-cell help is not present at the time of B-cell hyperactivity. Whether such decreased T-cell help precedes the B-cell hyperactivity is unknown; however, it does not appear to be likely. On the basis of in vitro studies, therefore, one would have to attribute the B-cell hyperactivity to abnormal responsiveness of the B cells to a greater extent than to excessive help from the T cells (Table 1-4).

In addition to helper T-cell function, suppressor T-cell function could be abnormal and fail to hold in check the excessive B-cell activity. A number of studies have attempted to demonstrate impaired suppressor T-cell function. Many papers have been written that demonstrate that patients with SLE have impaired Con A-induced T-suppressor function.[28] Even when such has been reported, however, the individual patients differ among themselves with regard to this type of defect; moreover, some patients have a defect for one function and not another.[81] As a result, there appears to be a substantial functional heterogeneity. Others have claimed that there is no such defect, largely by calling to question the Con A-induced suppressor system.[82] This may be a premature negation, since defects in suppressor function in SLE may be observed in the absence of Con A.[83] In addition, the immune system is more complex than simply having helper and suppressor cells. It appears that inducer cells are necessary for suppressor cells to become functional. Thus, $T4^+$ inducer cells are necessary to activate $T8^+$ suppressor-cell precursors to become suppressor-effector cells.[84,85] As a result, in SLE, a patient could have a defect in $T8^+$ cells (at the precursor or effector stage) and could have impaired function. Alternatively, a patient may have impaired inducer cells. In the absence of adequate $T4^+$ suppressor–inducer function, suppressor function would be impaired even with an intact $T8^+$ suppressor system. In fact, recent studies suggest that patients with SLE may be quite heterogeneous in terms of the T-cell defects they manifest. Some of this may not represent a primary problem but may be secondary to anti-T-cell antibodies that are produced by patients with SLE.

Consistent with the possibility that SLE patients may have different functional abnormalities is the observation that some patients with SLE may have high, low, or normal rations of $T4^+$ to $T8^+$ cells.[86] Those with high ratios appear to have different clinical features than those with low ratios.[86,87] Thus, SLE may not be a single illness in which we can hope to find a single mechanism of cellular dysfunction. Rather, it may be a syndrome with different cellular bases. Different individuals, therefore, may have different T-cell dysfunctions.

Another type of T-cell subdivision is a subdivision into T cells that bind autologous erythrocytes (Tar) and those that do not. The ability to bind autologous RBC appears not to relate to any kind of self-recognition, since heterologous RBC are bound as well as are autologous RBC.[88] Nevertheless, the cells that bind human RBC do seem to have special functional properties. These Tar cells are highly enriched in a suppressor function.[83,89,90] Moreover, anti-T-cell antibodies from patients with active SLE may preferentially eliminate such cells and their function.[83,91] As a result, it appears that anti-T-cell antibodies may be important in many of the functional abnormalities in SLE T-cell populations.

In addition to impaired helper and suppressor functions, SLE T cells appear to be inadequate in other areas. Patients with active SLE have markedly impaired dermal responses to recall antigens[68,92–94] and have impaired sensitization.[68,95,96] Since SLE patients manifest circulating T-cell lymphopenia,[28] it is possible that these deficiencies merely reflect reduced numbers of T cells. We (unpublished) and others[97] have observed restoration of many skin test responses following low-dose oral immunosuppressive drug treatment; this suggests that part of the impairment is due to suppressor efforts that are counteracted by the drugs. The dermal response to tuberculin, however, is impaired even in relatively inactive patients with reasonable lymphocyte numbers; this suggests a more severe abnormality.[28] In fact, studies have demonstrated a specific defect in responsiveness to mycobacteria.[98]

Recent advances in cellular immunology have emphasized that many of the cell interactions observed over the past 15 and more years do not arise from cells touching each other but, rather, result from the first cell elaborating a soluble factor that is able to bind to a receptor on the second cell so as to trigger it. The factors that are produced by lymphocytes are called *lymphokines* and those that are produced by monocytes are called *monokines*. These factors appear to be abnormally produced by the cells from many SLE patients. Thus, SLE patients have abnormally increased production of interferon[99–101] and impaired production of the monokine IL 1 and the lymphokine IL 2.[102,103] Since these latter factors are necessary for normal T cell activation and function, it is likely that some of the defects ascribed to the T cells of SLE patients may have a biochemical basis in a deficiency of adequate stimulatory signals. Since antibodies to interferon have been described in SLE,[104] it is possible that some of these deficiencies result from, rather than cause, autoimmune problems.

Anti-T Cell Antibodies

Initially viewed as a curiosity, these antibodies were subsequently held responsible for many abnormalities of SLE T cells, again exonerated, and more recently again held accountable. Patients with SLE make a great variety of autoantibodies, some of which react with leukocytes. Some of these are specific for T lymphocytes or their subsets. The most easily demonstrated anti-T cell antibodies are cold, reactive IgM antibodies. These have been shown to be capable of specifically eliminating T cells necessary for suppressor function.[105,106] It has been argued, however, that at body temperature such antibodies would not be able to have any effect. This argument is specious. Although the IgM antibodies may not induce C-mediated lysis at body temperature, they could certainly alter T cell recirculation patterns[77] and cause the T cells to be eliminated by the reticuloendothelial system. This problem has been largely resolved by the discovery of IgG anti-T-cell antibodies that are capable of eliminating suppressor function by the mechanism of antibody-dependent direct cellular cytotoxicity (ADCC).[92,107] Since this is a likely mechanism for tissue injury in many immune mediated diseases, such antibodies could plausibly be capable of eliminating T cells in vivo.

In addition to the initial studies that demonstrate that SLE anti-T cell antibodies are capable of eliminating suppressor T cell function, it has been found that such antibodies may preferentially kill Tar cells and eliminate their suppressor function[84,92,108] and that an SLE antibody may eliminate T-cell suppressor–inducer (T4) cells or suppressor–effector (T8) cells with resulting impaired suppressor function for Ig synthesis.[109] This finding provides two mechanisms by which anti-T cell antibodies could interfere with suppressor function and allow unhindered Ig synthesis as well as resolving the problem of some of the antibodies that react with T4 cells. Since Ia^+ T cells tend preferentially to include $T8^+$ cells and Tg cells,[110,111] it is possible that anti-Ia antibodies found in patients with SLE may contribute to a selective loss of T cell subsets. In addition, anti-Ia antibodies could prevent T cell activation in vivo; this thereby helps to explain impaired T-cell functions in general.

Natural Killer Cells

Natural killer cell are cells that are related to T cells by virtue of surface membrane characteristics and the ability to kill target cells. Unlike cytotoxic T cells, natural killer (NK) cells do not require prior sensitization to the target cell determinants in order to kill it. Unlike cells that mediate ADCC, the NK cell does not require the target cell to be coated by antibody. Nevertheless, the exact interrelationships between NK activity, ADCC, and cytotoxic T cells remain to be worked out. Of special note, NK cells appear to be unusual in having a positive feedback loop in which pre-NK cells are induced to become NK cells in the presence of interferon and the resulting cells produce interferon so as to recruit more NK cells from precursors.[112] This phenomenon is of special interest in SLE, since many patients during the course of active disease spontaneously produce large amounts of interferon.[99–101]

Patients with SLE have been reported to be deficient in NK activity.[113] This is somewhat surprising in view of the increase in interferon produced by many patients with SLE. A careful analysis by Katz et al.[113] has demonstrated, however, that patients with SLE have a defect in NK activity that is secondary to a deficiency in their capacity of NK cells to kill bound target cells. Since interferon is known to make target cells more resistant to such NK killing, increased interferon (IFN) production by SLE cells could be one explanation. Effects of anti-lymphocyte antibodies, previously reported to interfere with NK activity in SLE,[113] were not found in that study to interfere. Of interest, only the patients with active disease were found to be defective; those with inactive disease had normal NK activity.[113]

NK cells are known to be well endowed with F_c receptors that are capable of binding immune complexes. The association of increased disease activity and decreased NK function could possibly reflect the binding of immune complexes of NK cells and resultant decreased function.[113] Nevertheless, two studies specifically investigated this possibility and excluded it.[113] Not appreciated is the possibility that the most efficient NK cells were already inactivated and eliminated in vivo. This point was raised, however, by another group who reported that patients with SLE had a decrease in NK activity, which correlated with disease activity and also impaired augmentation of NK activity by IFN and virus-induced IFN.[114] Moreover, patients sometimes showed a dissociation among these functions, this suggested that the NK cells might have one or more defects in different patients. The failure of SLE NK cells to be stimulated by IFN[114,115] is reminiscent of the failure of SLE T cells and B cells to be easily stimulated in vitro (see above). A recent study has confirmed the impaired NK activity in patients with active SLE as well as in patients followed serially[116]. In addition, the NK cells failed to respond well to IFN inducers, even if the baseline NK activity was in the normal range. They found a normal ability of SLE cells to form effector target conjugates; however, the SLE NK cells failed adequately to produce a soluble cytotoxic factor necessary for lysis of the target. Whatever the mechanism of decreased NK activity in patient with active SLE, this deficit could provide another reason for increased susceptibility to certain types of infections in patients with active disease.

The Autologous Mixed Lymphocyte Reaction

T lymphocytes from normal people are capable of mounting a vigorous proliferative response when co-cultured with allogeneic non-T cells (cells from unrelated individuals). This reaction is called the "mixed lymphocyte reaction" and is conveniently studied by treating the stimulatory population in such a manner that it cannot contribute to the reaction being observed. Patients with SLE often manifest a defect in this reaction, especially when the disease is active.[117–119]

A somewhat related reaction is the responsiveness of T cells to stimulation by autologous non-T cells, called the "autologous mixed lymphocyte reaction" (AMLR). The AMLR has been demonstrated in both experimental animal and human cell systems; however, it has often been regarded as a curious reaction. Morever, a substantial controversy has existed regarding its existence in view of the presence of foreign materials (xenogeneic erythrocytes or fetal bovine serum or antibodies) used in cell separations or to support the culture growth. Most workers in the field not only believe that the AMLR is real but also that it provides an important insight into normal cell–cell interactions. This reaction, moreover, is defective in murine lupus[120–122] and in many immune-mediated diseases.

In the AMLR, T cells proliferate in response to autologous non-T cells. The proliferating T cells are of the $T4^+$ and the $T8^+$ phenotype; however, the $T8^+$ cells require help from the $T4^+$ cells.[123–125] This help can be replaced by IL 2.[123,126] The proliferating cells ultimately can provide help or suppression for Ig synthesis and mount cytotoxic reactions.[127–132] Thus, the reaction represents a mirror of normal cell–cell interactions, which might be operative in vivo. These interactions are known to be defective in patients with active SLE. Indeed, so is the AMLR.[133–136] Patients with very active disease were found to be uniformly defective, whereas those with less active disease were progressively less defective.[133,134] Moreover, the defect in the AMLR correlated with a defect in suppressor T-cell function.[133] Several additional studies have demonstrated the defect in patients with SLE and the correlation with disease activity, even in serially studied individual patients.[134]

Attempts to determine whether the defect in the AMLR was due to a responder T-cell defect or to a stimulatory non-T-cell defect suggested that either or both might be defective.[136,137] It appeared that patients with active disease had a defect in two different responding T-cell populations, whereas those with inactive or mildly active disease had a defect in only a single T-cell subset.[137] Additionally, active patients had defects in stimulatory non-T cells.[136,137] Since those studies, advances have been made in analyses of the AMLR, several of which are important to the SLE story: (i) different non-T cells vary in their stimulatory capacity[30,138] and (ii) the magnitude of the AMLR is itself regulated by T cells and macrophages, either of which can suppress the reaction but both together suppress best.[126] As a result, the AMLR in SLE recently has been reexamined.

It has been found that patients with active SLE have cells that in vitro have reduced IL 2 production and reduced IL 2 receptors on T4 cells (but normal IL 2 receptors on T8 cells). The T4 cells, therefore, do not make IL 2 and do not proliferate. IL 2 addition corrects the T4–T8 interactions because there are normal receptors on the T8 cells; however, exogenous IL 2 does not correct T4–T4 interactions because of the defect in IL 2 receptors on the T4 cells.[139] In addition, patients with different defects have differential responses to different stimuli; this suggests that the cellular basis for immune defects in different patients with SLE may be different.[140]

Monoclonal Autoantibodies: Clues to the Pathogenesis of SLE

Studies of monoclonal autoantibodies address questions of specificity. In addition, there is often an attempt to estimate the spectrum of autoantibody populations by immortalizing large numbers of individual B cells and studying the specificities of the immunoglobulin molecules produced. Distinct but related questions have been raised by such studies: (1) Can heterogeneous diseases be grouped on the basis of common reactivities, albeit in different organs? (2) Is the basis for heterogeneous autoantibody reactivities in the sera of patients really less complicated and less polyclonal than previously thought?

The question of the determinants with which a single monoclonal antibody might react is a recurring one. It has long been known that murine T lymphocytes share a determinant found in the brain. Reactivity of a single monoclonal antibody with apparently unrelated ligands has been demonstrated on several occasions.[141-144] A monoclonal autoantibody has been found to react with both human immunoglobulin and DNA histone.[55] Other monoclonal autoantibodies react with both DNA and cardiolipin, apparently by virtue of similar spacing of phosphodiester groups.[56,57] In both cases, the dual recognition represents "cross-reactivity." Such findings help to explain some of the unusual properties of antibodies previously observed in patients with autoimmune rheumatic diseases; they also help to define the specificities of the antibodies. Such studies, however, provide only minimal information with regard to the question of autoantibody heterogeneity in patients with autoimmune diseases. The finding that the nonautoimmune organisms can produce such monoclonal autoantibodies[58] demonstrates that it may be possible for an organism to have B cells capable of producing autoantibodies, but that such autoantibodies ordinarily are not produced in large amounts because of regulatory processes.[1] In other words, it is extremely difficult to extrapolate from either cross-reactive monoclonal autoantibodies or the spectrum of hybridoma monoclonal autoantibodies to the number of different clones of B cells involved in autoantibody production in vivo. Included among the difficulties are technical ones whereby some B cells more readily fuse and grow under the in vitro conditions. Whereas most anti-DNA molecules in the serum of patients are IgG, the anti-DNA hybridomas produced from such patients are preferentially IgM.[145]

It has been suggested that studies of monoclonal autoantibodies might yield information regarding the "immunogen(s)" responsible for autoantibody production. In cases of modified self-immunization, or immunization with a microbial (or viral) agent that cross-reacts with self determinants, such an analysis could conceivably provide useful clues. On the other hand, in such cases it is very likely that the autoantibody specificity bears very little relationship to the "immunogen" or represents only a small determinant on a larger structure from which one could easily deduce the whole.[146] Finally, when autoantibody production reflects polyclonal B-cell activation primarily and the specific expansion of subsets of B cells only secondarily, analysis of specificity may bypass certain critical pathogenetic mechanisms.[1]

GENETIC FEATURES OF HUMAN SYSTEMIC LUPUS ERYTHEMATOSUS

Human systemic lupus does not appear to be inherited as a single dominant trait. Far less than 50 percent of the offspring of affected individuals ultimately develop SLE. It is clear, nevertheless, that a predisposition to develop SLE can be inherited.[147,148] The concordance of disease in identical twins is greater than 67 percent (unpublished observations),[149] whereas dizygotic twins are at no greater risk than are other first-degree relatives.[149] Family studies indicate that relatives of patients with SLE have a much greater chance of developing the disease than do people in the general population.[147] Certain North American Indian tribes have a marked increase in SLE[150] and blacks develop the disease more readily than do Caucasians in the United States.[151] These larger populations augment the family studies in pointing to a genetic mechanism, although environmental factors could conceivably explain such clustering. The latter worry is illustrated by the lack of concordance of SLE in more than 30 percent of identical twins with the disease.[148]

Recent family studies have helped to clarify the genetic patterns.[152–154] These studies have provided evidence for aspects of the genetic bases for SLE already appreciated in studies of murine lupus: a single dominant or codominant gene can predispose to anti-DNA antibodies,[10,152] disease is inherited in a multigenic fashion,[12,154] and a subset of patients with SLE inherits an accelerating factor on the Y chromosome from the father.[1,2,4,153] It is thus possible that different patterns of inheritance may be associated with disease in the two sexes. Moreover, as in mice, it is likely that early in life disease may be inherited differently from late-life (middle-age) lupus. The former may require requisite "background" genes but may be mediated primarily by a single gene. This is probably the explanation for the Y chromosome-linked inheritance as well as the occurrence of disease in some of the females of those families (Table 1-3).

What could the genes for predisposition to lupus be? Obviously no answer is currently available; nevertheless, it is worth considering some of the possibilities. If antinuclear antibodies represent an important aspect of disease, an immune response gene for anti-DNA might be inherited as a single dominant or codominant gene. Alternatively, if DNA metabolic abnormalities are largely responsible for anti-DNA production by virtue of the release of especially immunogenic DNA,[155] gene(s) that code for an enzyme or other defect in this pathway (e.g., in DNA repair) could appear to act as genes for anti-DNA. In addition, abnormal estrogen metabolism reported in patients with SLE[156] might be inherited as a single gene; such a gene would be one of the background genes, which would augment immune responses, decrease immune regulation, and predispose to heightened autoantibody responses. A defect in normal suppressor-cell function could be inherited as one of many background genes that predispose to SLE. Evidence for such a process has been put forth in families of SLE patients.[157] Since not all of those affected by the defect had autoimmune disease, it appears that additional genes (or a critical environment influence) would be necessary. A defect in immune regulation that leads to excessive B-cell activation, thus, might come about by any of several abnormalities in the immune system; the genes that code for any of these defects would serve as "background" genes, which predispose to SLE.

So far, nothing has been mentioned of the major histocompatibility types of patients with SLE. Although much has been made of disease associations with HLA types, the relative risks associated with SLE and HLA-D3 and HLA-D2 are models.[158] It is likely that a gene associated with HLA-D3 predisposes to increased antibody responses and decreased antigen clearance and thereby predisposes to "immune complex" and antibody-mediated diseases.[159] A most interesting association is that of SLE and decrease numbers of C3b receptors on erythrocytes.[160] Rather than representing an immune-response gene, this form of inheritance probably decreases the clearance of injurious antibodies and antigen–antibody complexes and thereby predisposes to disease. A variety of "background" genes, thus, can predispose to SLE. The more of these genes that are found in a given individual, the more likely disease would be expressed. On the other hand, a single gene in mice can entirely or largely prevent the expression of autoimmunity and the development of lupus.[1,16–164] Whether such protective genes are present in humans is unknown. The presence of such genes could help to explain some of the incomplete penetrance observed in family studies. In addition, knowledge of such genes could help family planning and also help approaches to therapy.

SYNTHESIS

Is it possible to put the above information together so as to shed light upon pathogenetic events in SLE? A complete picture cannot be drawn; however, some of the outlines fall into place. Since SLE may be genetically and clinically heterogeneous, it is likely that we are dealing with a syndrome rather than a single disease. This is, in some measure, a semantic matter; however, if we recognize that the basis for disease might be different in different individuals, it allows us better to deal with diversity of biological abnormalities as well as diversity in clinical manifestations.

The central aspect of SLE is a predisposition of B cells to proliferate and differentiate into immunoglobulin-secreting cells. Patients must, therefore, have an abnormality that leads to excessive B-cell proliferation and differentiation. This abnormality might be an inherited defect. The precise defect might be different in different individuals, some having excess stimulation of the B cells, some having impaired regulation of the B cells, and some having excessively activatable B cells. In some individuals, excessive production of B cells from stem cells might be an underlying problem. Finally, some patients may have no major inherited predisposition to B-cell hyperactivity but might be stimulated sufficiently by exogenous sources to yield disease.

The second major abnormality of patients with SLE is that they produce particular kinds of autoantibodies. Although patients may produce a great variety of autoantibodies, antibodies reactive with DNA and other nuclear antigens are especially characteristic. Of interest, nucleic acids are capable of acting as immune adjuvants. It is therefore possible for a nucleic acid to act both as an immunogen and as a polyclonal immune activator in patients. It may, however, require the appropriate second kind of gene, one that either leads to a biochemical abnormality of nucleic acid metabolism or one that allows a vigorous immune response to nucleic acid antigens or some antigen that induces antibodies that cross-react with DNA. In this regard, we should recognize that the antibodies produced to self-antigens could actually be induced by cross-reactive immunogens that bear only a modest relationship to the self-antigens.[59]

The process of polyclonal immune activation leads to a great variety of secondary phenomena. These are most of the phenomena we measure when we study cells from patients with active SLE. They include spontaneous B-cell hyperactivity but impaired B-cell responses to in vitro stimuli and impaired in vivo and in vitro T-cell functions of many kinds, many related to a decrease in necessary growth factor production as well as suppression as a result of the in vivo immune activation and a form of endogenous antigenic competition. Finally, antilymphocyte antibodies, immune complexes, etc. act to interfere further with normal immunoregulatory processes. The activated immune system leads to in vivo interferon production and further resistance to interferon-mediated phenomena, this includes NK activity, in vitro.

How does this process get triggered? It should be clear that studying the full-blown process provides one with many abnormalities, some of which are very important in disease production and many of which are important in perpetuating the defective state but very few of which initiated the process. Possible triggers are endogenous metabolic abnormalities and exogenous stimuli. Among the latter, viral infections, which induce interferon production, could initiate the process. Bacterial infections, which induce DR expression by macrophages, also could initiate the process. Additional agents, which mimic the various growth factors, also are capable of pushing the immune system toward increased activity. Ultraviolet light acts as a trigger in some individuals. Two explanations readily present themselves: DNA alteration and interference with macrophage functions. Ultraviolet light is capable of altering the structure of DNA; such an alteration might make it especially good at inducing either polyclonal immune activation of anti-DNA production. This is especially so in the face of impaired DNA repair in SLE. Less well appreciated is the profound suppressive effect of ultraviolet light on the ability of macrophages to handle antigens. This effect could have an adverse effect remote from the skin. A critical feature is failure of the system to turn itself off once the process is initiated. A perpetual anti-self-immune reaction is thus possible. Only by interfering with the immune circuitry can we bring the entire process to an end. From a therapeutic point of view, it might be possible to allow the immune defects to continue and merely eliminate the final common pathway: autoantibody production or its consequences. It thus might be possible to eliminate the B cells that make autoantibodies[161–164] or reduce the impact of mediator release[165,166] and thereby bring about a useful end result without altering the fundamental processes. With the advent of modern immunotechnology, novel approaches to the therapy of SLE and other immune-mediated diseases are moving from the realm of fantasy to the arena of possibility.

REFERENCES

1. Smith HR, Steinberg AD: Autoimmunity: A perspective. Ann Rev Immunol 1:175–210, 1983
2. Theofilopolous AN, Dixon FJ: Etiopathogenesis of murine systemic lupus erythematosus. Immunol Rev 55:179–216, 1981
3. Steinberg AD, Huston DP, Taurog JD, et al.: The cellular and genetic basis of murine lupus. Immunol Rev 55:121–154, 1981
4. Murphy ED: Lymphoproliferation (LPR) and other single-locus models for murine lupus, in Gershwin ME, Merchant B, (eds): Immunologic Defects in Laboratory Animals. New York, Plenum, 1981
5. Eisenberg RA, Dixon FJ: Effect of castration on male-determined acceleration of autoimmune disease in BXSB mice. J Immunol 125:1959–1961, 1980
6. Delfraissy JF, Segond P, Galanaud P, et al.: Depressed primary in vitro antibody response in untreated systemic lupus erythematosus: T helper cell defect and lack of defective suppressor cell function. J Clin Invest 66:141, 1980
7. Morse HC III, Davidson WF, Yetter RA, et al.: Abnormalities induced by the mutual gene *lpr:* Expansion of a unique lymphocyte subset. J Immunol 129:2612, 1982
8. Steinberg AD, Melez KA, Raveche ES, et al.: Approach to the study of the role of sex hormones in autoimmunity. Arthritis Rheum 22:1170–1176, 1979
9. Roubinian JR, Talal N, Greenspan JS, et al.: Effect of castration and sex hormone treatment on survival antinucleic acid antibodies, and glomerulonephritis in NZB/NZW F_1 mice. J Exp Med 147:1568–1581, 1978
10. Raveche ES, Steinberg AD, Klassen LW, et al.: Genetic studies in NZB mice. I. Spontaneous autoantibody production. J Exp Med 147:1487–1502, 1978
11. Yoshida H, Kohno A, Ohta K, et al.: Genetic studies of autoimmunity in New Zealand Mice. III. Associations among anti-DNA antibodies, NTA, and renal disease in NZB × NZW F_1 × NZW backcross mice. J Immunol 127:433–437, 1981
12. Raveche ES, Novotny EA, Hansen CT, et al.: Genetic studies in NZB mice. V. Recombinant inbred lines demonstrate that separate genes control autoimmune phenotype. J Exp Med 153:1187—1197, 1981
13. Dixon FJ, Oldstone MBA, Tonietti G: Pathogenesis of immune complex glomerulonephritis of New Zealand mice. J Exp Med 134:65s–71s, 1971
14. Mellors RC, Shiari T, Aoki T: Wildtype gross leukemia virus and the pathogenesis of the glomerulonephritis of New Zealand mice. J Exp Med 133:113–126, 1971
15. Datta SD, Owne FL, Womack JE, et al.: Analysis of recombinant inbred lines derived from "autoimmune" (NZB) and "high leukemia" (C58) strains: Independent multigenic systems control B cell hyperactivity, retrovirus expression, and autoimmunity. J Immunol 129:1539–1544, 1982
16. Tonietti G, Oldstone MB, Dixon FJ: The effect of induced chronic viral infections on the immunologic diseases of New Zealand mice. J Exp Med 132:89–109, 1970
17. Steinberg AD, Roths JB, Murphy ED, et al.: Effects of thymectomy or andro-

gen administration upon the autoimmune disease of MRL/MP-1pr/1pr mice. J Immunol 125:871–873, 1980
18. Smith HR, Chused TM, Smathers PA, et al.: Evidence for thymic regulation of autoimmunity in BXSB mice: Acceleration of disease by neonatal thymectomy. J Immunol 130:1200–1204, 1983
19. Ranney DF, Steinberg AD: Differences in the age-dependent release of a low molecular weight suppressor (LMWS) and stimulators by normal and NZB/W lymphoid organs. J Immunol 117:1219–1225, 1976
20. Morton JI, Siegel BV: Transplantation of autoimmune potential. I. Development of antinuclear antibodies in H-2 histocompatible recipients of bone marrow from New Zealand black mice. Proc Natl Acad Sci USA 71:2162–2165, 1974
21. Morton JI, Siegal BV: Transplantation of autoimmune potential. III. Immunological hyper-responsiveness and elevated endogenous spleen colony formation in lethally irradiated recipients of NZB bone marrow cells. Immunology 34:863–868, 1978
22. Eisenberg RA, Izui S, McConahey PF, et al.: Male determined accelerated autoimmune disease in BXSB mice: Transfer by bone marrow and spleen cells. J Immunol 125:1032–1036, 1980
23. Akizuki M, Reeves JP, Steinberg AD: Expression of autoimmunity by NZB/NZW marrow. Clin Immunol Immunopathol 10:247–250, 1978
24. Denman AM, Russell AS, Denman EJ: Adoptive transfer of the disease of NZB mice to normal mouse strains. Clin Exp Immunol 5:567, 1969
25. Theofilopoulos AN, Balderas RS, Shawler DL, et al.: Influence of thymic genotype on the systemic lypus erythematosus—like disease and T cell proliferation of mr1/Mp-1pr mice. J Exp Med 153:1405–1414, 1981
26. Laskin CA, Smathers PA, Reeves JP, et al.: Studies of defective tolerance induction in NZB mice: Evidence for a marrow pre-T cell defect. J Exp Med 155:1025–136, 1982
27. Hang L, Izui S, Slack JH, et al.: The cellular basis for resistance to induction of tolerance in BXSB systemic lupus erythematosus male mice. J Immunol 129:787–789, 1982
28. Raveche ES, Steinberg AD: Lymphocytes and lymphocyte functions in systemic lupus erythematosus. Clin Haematol 15:344–370, 1979
29. Glinski W, Gershwin ME, Budman DR, et al.: Study of lymphocyte subpopulations in normal humans and patients with systemic lupus erythematosus by fractionation of peripheral blood lymphocytes on a discontinuous ficoll gradient. Clin Exp Immunol 26:228–238, 1976
30. Smolen JS, Sharrow SO, Reves JP, et al.: The human autologous mixed lymphocyte reaction: Suppression by macrophages and T cells. J Immunol 127:1987–1993, 1981
31. Kirchner H, Fernbach BR, Herberman RB: Macrophages suppressing T and B cell mitogen responses and the mixed leukocyte reaction, in Oppenheim JJ, Rosenstreich DL, (eds.): Mitogens in Immunology, New York, Academic Press, 1976
32. Cass RM, Mongan ES, Jacox-Vaughan JH: Immunoglobulins G, A, and M in systemic lupus erythematosus. Ann Intern Med 69:749–756, 1968
33. Claman HN, Merrill D: Quantitative measurement of human $gamma_2$ and $beta_{2m}$ serum immunoglobulins. J Lab Clin Med 64:685, 1964
34. Harvey AM, Schulman LE, Tumulty PA, et al.: Systemic lupus erthematosus: Review of the literature and analysis of 138 cases. Medicine (Baltimore) 33:291–437, 1954
35. Quismorio FP, Friou GJ: Serological factors in systemic lupus erythematosus and their pathogenetic significance. CRC Crit Rev Clin Lab Sci 639–683, 1970
36. Onodera S: Quantitative determination of serum immunoglobulins in various diseases. Tohoku J Exp Med 89:279, 1966
37. Lee SL, Meiselas LE, Zingale SB, et al.: Antibody production in systemic lupus erythematosus (SLE) and rheumatoid arthritis (RA). J Clin Invest 39:1005–1006, 1960
38. Levy J, Barnett EV, MacDonald NS, et al.: Altered immunoglobulin metabolism in systemic lupus erythematosus

and rheumatoid arthritis. J Clin Invest 49:708–715, 1970
39. Delbarre F, Pompidou A, Kahan A, et al.: Study of blood lymphocytes during systemic lupus erythematosus. Pathol Biol (Paris) 19:379–387, 1971
40. Delbarre F, Go LA, Kahan A: Hyperbasophilic immunoblasts in the circulating blood in chronic inflammatory rheumatoic and collagen diseases. Ann Rheum Dis 34:422–430, 1975
41. Marmont AM, Damasio E: Circulating hyperbasophilic mononuclear cells in systemic lupus erythematosus, in Linder J, Ruttner J, Miescher P, et al (eds): Arthritis-Arthrose. Bern, Stuttgart, Wein, Verlag Hans Huber, 1971
42. Michael SR, Yural IL, Basson VA, et al.: The hematologic aspects of disseminated (systemic) lupus erythematosus patients. Blood 6:1059–1072, 1951
43. Jasin HE, Ziff M: Immunoglobulin synthesis by peripheral blood cells in systemic lupus erythematosus. Arthritis Rheum 18:219, 1975
44. Ginsburg WW, Finkelman FD, Lipsky PE: Circulating and pokeweed mitogen-induced immunoglobulin-secreting cells in systemic lupus erythematosus. Clin Exp Immunol 35:76–88, 1979
45. Blaese RM, Grayson J, Steinberg AD: Elevated immunoglobulin secreting cells in the blood of patients with active systemic lupus erythematosus: Correlation of laboratory and clinical assessment of disease activity. Am J Med 69:345–350, 1980
46. Wangel AG, Milton A, Egan JB: Spontaneous plaque forming cells in the peripheral blood of patients with systemic lupus erythematosus. Clin Exp Immunol 49:41–49, 1982
47. Tan PLJ, Pang GTM, Cullinane G, et al.: Immunoglobulin secreting cells in SLE: Correlation with disease activity. J Rheumatol 7:807–813, 1980
48. Tan P, Pang G, Wilson JD: Immunoglobulin production in vitro by peripheral blood lymphocytes in systemic lupus erythematosus: Helper T cell defect and B cell hyperreactivity. Clin Exp Immunol 44:548–554, 1981
49. Okudaira K, Tanimoto K, Nakamura T, et al.: Spontaneously enhanced in vitro immunoglobulin synthesis by bulls in systemic lupus erythematosus. Clin Immunol Immunopathol 16:267, 1980
50. Tsokos GC, Balow JE: Spontaneous and pokeweed mitogen-induced plaque-forming cells in systemic lupus erythematosus. Clin Immunol Immunopathol 21:172–183, 1981
51. Steinberg AD, Smolen JS, Sakane T, et al.: Immune regulatory abnormalities in systemic lupus erythematosus, Cummings N, Michael A, Wilson C, (eds): in Immune Mechanisms of Renal Disease, New York, Plenum Press, 1983
52. Fauci AS, Steinberg AD, Haynes BF, et al.: Immunoregulatory aberrations in systemic lupus erythematosus. J Immunol 121:1473–1479, 1978
53. Budman DR, Merchant EB, Steinberg AD, et al.: Increased spontaneous activity of antibody-forming cells in the peripheral blood of patients with active SLE. Arth Rheum 20:829–833, 1977
54. Morimoto C, Abe T, Hara M, et al.: In vitro TNP-specific antibody formation by peripheral lymphocytes from patients with systemic lupus erythematosus. Scand J Immunol 6:575–579, 1977
55. Agnello V, Arbetter A, Ibanez de Kaspep G, et al.: J Exp Med 151:1514, 1981
56. Shoenfeld Y, Rauch J, Massicotte H, et al.: N Engl J Med 308:414, 1983
57. Lafter EM, Rauch J, Andrzejewski C, et al.: J Exp Med 153:897, 1981
58. Haspel MV, Onodera T, Prabhakar BS, et al.: Nature 304:73–76, 1983
59. Steinberg AD: Actiology of autoimmunity. Nature 304:20, 1983
60. Steinberg AS, Kaltreider HB, Staples PJ, et al.: Cyclophosphamide in lupus nephritis: A controlled trial. Ann Intern Med 75:165–171, 1971
61. Bobrove AM, Miller P: Depressed in vitro B-lymphocyte differentiation in systemic lupus erythematosus. Arthritis Rheum 20:1326–1333, 1977
62. Brodman R, Gilfillan R, Glass D, et al.: Influenza vaccine response in systemic lupus erythematosus. Ann Intern Med 88:735–740, 1978
63. Louie JS, Nies KM, Shoji KT, et al.: Clinical and antibody responses after influenza immunization in systemic lupus

erythematosus. Ann Intern Med 88:790–792, 1978
64. Ristow SC, Douglas RC, Condemi JJ: Influenza vaccination of patients with systemic lupus erythematosus. Ann Intern Med 88:786–789, 1978
65. Williams GW, Steinberg AD, Reinertsen JL, et al.: Influenza immunization in systemic lupus erythematosus: A double-blind trial. Ann Intern Med 88:729–734, 1978
66. Baum J, Ziff M: Decreased 19S antibody response to bacterial antigens in systemic lupus erythematosus. J Clin Invest 48:758–767, 1969
67. Abe T, Homma M: Immunological reactivity in patients with systemic lupus erythematosus (humoral antibody and cellular immune response). Acta Rheum Scand 17:35–46, 1971
68. Muschel LW: Systemic lupus erythematosus and normal antibodies. Proc Soc Exp Biol Med 106:622–625, 1961
69. Zingale SB, Sanchez AJC, Andrada JA, et al.: Appearance of anticoagulant factors and certain autoimmune antibodies following antigenic stimulation with blood group substances in patients with systemic lupus erythematosus. Arthritis Rheum 6:581–598, 1963
70. Harris J, Vaughan J: Penicillin antibody in disease. J Clin Invest 39:995, 1960
71. Evans AS, Rothfeld NF: Virus and other viral antibodies in systemic lupus erythematosus. Lancet 1:1127, 1973
72. Hollinger FB, Sharp JT, Lidsky MD, et al.: Antibodies to viral antigens in systemic lupus erythematosus. Arthritis Rheum 14:1–11, 1971
73. Hurd ER, Dowdle W, Casey H, et al.: Virus antibody levels in systemic lupus erythematosus. Arthritis Rheum 15:267–274, 1972
74. Phillips PE, Christian CL: Virus antibody studies in the connective tissue diseases. Arthritis Rheum 14:180–181, 1971
75. Wilson CB, Dixon FJ, Evans AS, et al.: Antiviral antibody responses in patients with renal disease. Clin Immunol Immunopathol 2:121–132, 1973
76. Pincus T, Steinberg AD, Blacklow N, et al.: Reactivities of systemic lupus erythematosus sera with cellular and virus antigen preparations. Arthritis Rheum 21:873–879, 1978
77. Gelfand MC, Parker LM, Steinberg AD: Mechanism of allograft rejection in New Zealand mice. II. Role of a serum factor. J Immunol 113:1–8, 1974
78. Adler FL: Competition of antigens. Prog Allergy 8:41, 1964
79. Glinski W, Gershwin ME, Steinberg AD: Fractionation of cells on a discontinuous Ficoll gradient: Study of subpopulations of human T cells using anti-T cell antibodies from patients with systemic lupus erythematosus. J Clin Invest 57:604–614, 1976
80. Kumagai S, Sredni B, House S, et al.: Defective regulation of B lymphocyte colony formation in patients with systemic lupus erythematosus. J Immunol 128:258–262, 1981
81. Sakane T, Steinberg AD, Green I: Studies of immune functions of patients with systemic lupus erythematosus. I. Failure of suppressor T cell activity related to impaired generation of, rather than response to, suppressor cells. Arth Rheum 21:657–664, 1978
82. Nakamura Z, Asano T, Yano K, et al.: Reevaluation of suppressor cell function in systemic lupus erythematosus. Clin Immunol Immunopathol 24:72–82, 1982
83. Kumagai S, Steinberg AD, Green I: Immune responses to hapten-modified self and their regulation in normal individuals and patients with SLE. J Immunol 127:1643–1652, 1981
84. Reinherz EL, Morimoto C, Fitzgerald KA, et al.: Heterogeneity of human $T4^+$ inducer T cells defined by a monoclonal antibody that delineates two functional subpopulations. J Immunol 128:463, 1982
85. Thomas Y, Rogozinski L, Irigoyen OH, et al.: Functional analysis of human T cell subsets defined by monoclonal antibodies. V. Suppressor cells within the activated $OKT4^+$ population belong to a distinct subset. J Immunol 128:1386, 1982
86. Smolen JS, Chused TM, Leiserson WM, et al.: Heterogeneity of immunoregulatory T cell subsets in systemic lupus ery-

thematosus: Correlation with clinical features. Am J Med 72:783–790, 1982.
87. Smolen JS, Morimoto C, Chused TM, et al.: T cell subsets in systemic lupus erythematosus (SLE): Correlation with clinical features. Arthritis Rheum 25s:36, 1982
88. Smolen JS, Sharrow SO, Steinberg AD: Characterization of autologous rosette forming cells: A non-restricted phenomenon. J Immunol 127:737–742, 1981
89. Palacios R, Alarcon-Segovia D, Llorente L, et al.: Human post-thymic precursor cells in health and disease. Immunology 42:127, 1981
90. Kumagai S, Scher I, Green I: Autologous rosette-forming T cells regulate responses of T cells: Phenotypic and functional analysis of suppressor cells generated from autologous rosette forming T cells after autologous mixed lymphocyte reactions. J Clin Invest 68:356, 1981
91. Kumagai S, Steinberg AD, Green I: Antibodies to T cells in patients with systemic lupus erythematosus mediated ADCC against human T cell. J Clin Invest 67:605–614, 1981
92. Andrianakos AA, Tsichlis PN, Merikas EG, et al.: Cell-mediated immunity in systemic lupus erythematosus. Clin Exp Immunol 30:89–96, 1977
93. Gottlieb AB, Lahita RG, Chiorazzi N, et al.: Immune function in systemic lupus erythematosus: Impairment of in vitro T-cell proliferation and in vivo antibody response to exogenous antigen. J Clin Invest 63:885–892, 1979
94. Hahn BH, Babgy MK, Osterland CK: Abnormalities of delayed hypersensitivity in systemic lupus erythematosus. Am J Med 55:25–31, 1973
95. Horwitz DA, Garrett MA: Lymphocyte reactivity to mitogens in subjects with systemic lupus erythematosus, rheumatoid arthritis and scleroderma. Clin Exp Immunol 27:92–99, 1977
96. Landry M: Phagocyte function and cell-mediated immunity in systemic lupus erythematosus. Arch Dermatol 113:147–154, 1977
97. Tripodi D, Parks LC, Brugmans J: Drug-induced restoration of cutaneous delayed hypersensitivity in anergic patients. N Engl J Med 289:354–359, 1973
98. Wadee AA, Gear AJ, Rabson AR: Production of a suppressor factor by human adherent cells treated with *Mycobacterium tuberculosis:* Absence in systemic lupus erythematosus. Clin Exp Immunol 46:82–88, 1981
99. Hooks JJ, Moutsopoulos HM, Geis SA, et al.: Immune interferon in the circulation of patients with autoimmune disease. N Engl J Med 301:5–8, 1979
100. Hooks JJ, Jordan GW, Gupps T, et al.: Multiple interferons in systemic lupus erythematosus and vasculitis. Arthritis Rheum 25:396–400, 1982
101. Ytterberg SR, Schnitzer TJ: Serum interferon levels in patients with systemic lupus erythematosus. Arthritis Rheum 25:401–406, 1982
102. Aloccer-Varela J, Alarcon-Segovia D: Decreased production of and response to interleukin 2 by cultured lymphocytes from patients with systemic lupus erythematosus. J Clin Invest 69:1388–1392, 1982
103. Horwitz DA, Linker-Israeli M, Bakke AC, et al.: Characterization of the mechanisms responsible for Interleukin 1 and 2 deficiencies in patients with systemic lupus erythematosus. Arthritis Rheum 26:s28, 1983
104. Panem S, Check IJ, Henriksen D, et al.: Antibodies to 06-interferon in a patient with system lupus erythematosus. J Immunol 129:1–3, 1982
105. Sakane T, Reeves JP, Steinberg AD, et al.: Studies of immune functions of patients with systemic lupus erythematosus: Complement dependent immunoglobulin M anti-thymus-derived cell antibodies preferentially inactive suppressor cells. J Clin Invest 63:954–965, 1979
106. Sakane T, Steinberg AD, Reeves JP, et al.: Studies of immune functions of patients with systemic lupus erythematosus: T cell subsets and antibodies to T cell subsets. J Clin Invest 64:1260–1269, 1979
107. Okudaira K, Searles RP, Tanimoto K, et al.: T-lymphocyte interaction with immunoglobulin G antibody in systemic lupus erythematosus. J Clin Invest 69:1026–1038, 1982

108. Green I, Kumagai S, Steinberg AD: Immune responses to hapten-modified self and their regulation in normal individuals and patients with SLE. Arthritis Rheum 25:824–827, 1982
109. Morimoto C, Reinherz EL, Steinberg AD, et al.: Relationship between SLE T cell subsets, anti-T cell antibodies, and T cell functions. Arthritis Rheum 26:s27, 1983
110. Kaszuhowski SA, Goodwin JS, Williams RC: Ia antigen on the surface of a subfraction of T cells that bear Fo receptors for IgG. J Immunol 124:1075–1078, 1980
111. Greaves MF, Verbi W, Festenstein H, et al.: "Ia-like" antigens on human T cells. Eur J Immunol 9:356–362, 1979
112. Silva A, Bonavida B, Targan S: Mode of action of interferon-mediated modulation of natural killer cytotoxic activity: Recruitment of pre NK cells and enhanced Kinetics of lysis. J Immunol 125: 479–484, 1980
113. Hoffman T: Natural killer function in systemic lupus erythematosus. Arthritis Rheum 23:30–31, 1980
114. Goto M, Tanimoto K, Horiuchi Y: Natural cell-mediated cytotoxicity in systemic lupus erythematosus. Suppression by antilymphocyte antibody. Arthritis Rheum 23:1274–1279, 1980
115. Karsh J, Dorval G, Osterland CK: Natural cytotoxicity in rheumatoid arthritis and systemic lupus erythematosus. Clin Immunol Immunopathol 19:437–448, 1981
116. Ytterberg SR, Huard TK, Schnitzer TJ: Effects of serum from patients with systemic lupus erythematosus on natural killer cell activity and antibody-dependent cell-mediated cytotoxicity. Clin Res 29:786A, 1981
117. Rook AH, Stocks N, Tsokos GC, et al.: Immunogobulin G autoantibodies to natural killer cells in systemic lupus erythematosus. Clin Res 29:488A, 1981
118. Katz P, Zaytoun AM, Lee Jr, JH, et al.: Abnormal natural killer cell activity in systemic lupus erythematosus: an intrinsic defect in the lytic event. J Immunol 129:1966–1971, 1982
119. Parrillo JE, Fauci AS: Comparison of the effector cells in human spontaneous cellular cytotoxicity and antibody-dependent cellular cytotoxicity: differential sensitivity of effector cells to in vivo and in vitro corticosteroids. Scand J Immunol 8:99–107, 1978
120. Neighbour PA, Grayzel AI, Miller AE: Endrogenous and interferon-augmented natural killer cell activity of human peripheral blood mononuclear cells in vitro. Studies of patients with multiple sclerosis, systemic lupus erythematosus or rheumatoid arthritis. Clin exp Immunol 49:11–21, 1982
121. Fitzharris P, Alcocer J, Stephens HA, et al.: Insensitivity to interferon of NK cells from patients with systemic lupus erythematosus. Clin exp Immunol 47:110–118, 1982
122. Sibbitt WL, Jr, Mathews PM, Bankhurst AD: Natural killer cell in systemic lupus erythematosus. J Clin Invest 71:1230–1239, 1983
123. Paty JG, Sienknecht CW, Townes AS, et al.: Impaired cell-mediated immunity in systemic lupus erythematosus. Am J Med 59:769–779, 1975
124. Suciu-Foca N, Buda JA, Thiem T, et al.: Impaired responsiveness of lymphocytes in patients with systemic lupus erythematosus. Clin Exp Immunol 18:295–301, 1974
125. Werne P, Kunkel HG: Antibodies to a specific surface antigen of T-cells in human sera inhibiting mixed leukocyte culture reactions. J Exp Med 138:1021–1026, 1973
126. Smith JB, Pasternak RD: Syngenic mixed leukocyte reaction in mice; strain distribution, kinetics, participating cells, and absence in NZB mice. J Immunol 122:1889, 1978
127. Glimcher LH, Steinberg AD, House SB, et al.: The autologous mixed lymphocyte reaction in strains of mice with autoimmune disease. J Immunol 125:1832–1838, 1980
128. Hom JT, Talal N: Decreased syngeneic mixed lymphocyte response in autoimmune susceptible mice. Scand J Immunol 15:195, 1982

129. Smolen JS, Luger TA, Chused TM, et al.: Responder cells in the human autologous mixed lymphocyte reaction. J Clin Invest 68:1601, 1981
130. Damle NK, Gupta S: Autologous mixed lymphocyte reaction in man. V. Functionally and phenotypically distinct human T-cell subpopulations respond to non-T and activated T cells in AMLR. Scand J Immunol 16:269, 1982
131. Palacios R, Moller G: HLA-DR antigens render resting T cells sensitive to interleukin 2 and induce production of the growth factor in the autologous mixed lymphocyte reaction. Cell Immunol 63:143–151, 1981
132. Smolen JS, Chused TM, Novotny EA, et al.: The human autologous mixed lymphocyte reaction. III. Immune circuits. J Immunol 129:1050, 1982
133. Weksler ME, Kozak R: Lymphocyte transformation induced by autologous cells. V. Generation of immunologic memory and specificity during the autologous mixed lymphocyte reaction. J Exp Med 146:1833, 1977
134. Stouwe RAV, Kunkel HG, Halper JP, et al.: Autologous mixed lymphocyte culture reactions and generation of cytotoxic T cells. J Exp Med 146:1809, 1977
135. Hausmann PB, Stobo JD: Specificity and function of human autologous reaction T cell. J Exp Med 149:1537, 1979
136. Sakane T, Green I: Specificity and suppressor function of human T cells responsive to autologous non-T cells. J Immunol 123:584, 1979
137. Shin HS, Wang CY, Choi YS: Activation of autologous reactive helper T lymphocytes for differentiation of human B lymphocytes. J Immunol 127:2485, 1981
138. Gatenby PA, Kotzin BL, Kansas CS, et al.: Immunoglobulin secretion in the human autologous mixed leucocyte reaction: Definition of a suppressor-amplifier circuit using monoclonal antibodies. J Exp Med 156:55, 1982
139. Sakane T, Steinberg AD, Green I: Failure of autologous mixed lymphocyte reactions between T and non-T cells in patients with systemic lupus erythematosus. Proc Natl Acad Sci USA 75:3464–3468, 1978
140. Sakane T, Steinberg AJ, Green I: Studies of immune functions of patients with systemic lupus erythematosus. V. T-cell suppressor function and autologous MLR during active and inactive phases of disease. Arthritis Rheum 23:225–231, 1980
141. Smith JB, DeHoratius RJ: Deficient autologous mixed reactions correlate with disease activity in systemic lupus erythematosus and rheumatoid arthritis. Clin Exp Immunol 48:155, 1982
142. Kuntz MM, Innes JB, Weksler ME: The cellular basis of the impaired autologous mixed lymphocyte reaction in patients with systemic lupus erythematosus. J Clin Invest 63:151, 1979
143. Sakane T, Steinberg AD, Arnett FC, et al.: Studies of immune functions of patients with systemic lupus erythematosus. III. Characterization of lymphocyte subpopulations responsible for defective autologous mixed lymphocyte reactions. Arthritis Rheum 22:770, 1979
144. Kuntz-Crow M, Kunkel HG: Human dendritic cells: Major stimulators of the autologous and allogeneic mixed leukocyte reactions. Clin Exp Immunol 49:338–350, 1982
145. Takada S, Murakawa Y, Ueda Y, et al.: Abnormalities in autologous mixed lymphocyte reaction-activated immune circuits in systemic lupus erythematosus and their possible correction by interkeukin 2. J Immunol (in press)
146. Smolen JS, Siminovitch K, Luger TA, et al.: Responder cells in the human autologous mixed lymphocyte reaction (AMLR). II. Characterization and interactions in healthy individuals and patients with systemic lupus erythematosus: Proceedings of the first international symposium on the AMLR. Behring Inst. M:H. 72:135–142, 1983
147. Lane DP, Hoeffler WK: SV40 large T shares an antigenic determinant with a cellular protein of molecular weight 68,000. Nature 288:167–170, 1980
148. Pillemer E, Weissman IL: A monoclonal antibody that detects a Vk-tepc15

idiotypic determinant cross-reactive with a thy-1 determinant. J Exp Med 153:1068–1079, 1981
149. Johnston MFM, Elsen HN: Cross-reactions between 2,-4 dinitrophenyl and menadione (vitamin K3) and the general problem of antibody specificity. J Immunol 117:1189–1196, 1976
150. Lane D, Koprowski H: Molecular recognition and the future of monoclonal antibodies. Nature 296:200–202, 1982
151. Shoenfeld Y, Hsu-Lin SC, Gabriels JE, et al.: Production of autoantibodies by human-human hybridomas. J Clin Invest 70:205–208, 1982
152. Wel van der H: Physiological action and structure characteristics of the sweet-tasting proteins thaumatin and monellin. Trends Biochem Sci 5:122–123, 1980
153. Arnett FC, Shulman LE: Studies in familial systemic lupus erythematosis. Medicine (Baltimore) 55:313–322, 1976
154. Block SR, Lockshin MD, Winfield JB, et al.: Immunological observations on 9 sets of twins either concordant or discordant for SLE. Arthritis Rheum 19:545–554, 1976
155. Raveche ES, Steinberg AD, Klassen LW, et al.: Genetic studies in NZB mice. I. Spontaneous autoantibody production. J Exp Med 147: 1487–1498, 1978
156. Morton RO, Gershwin ME, Brady C, et al.: Incidence of systemic lupus erythematosus (SLE) in North American Indians. J Rheumatol 3:186–190, 1976
157. Kaslow RA, Masi AT: Age, sex, and race effects on mortality from systemic lupus erythematosus in the United States, Arthritis Rheum 21:473–484, 1978
158. Lippman SM, Arnett FC, Conley CL, et al.: Genetic factors predisposing to autoimmune disease. Am J Med 73:827–840, 1982
159. Lahita RG, Chiorazzi N, Gibofsky A, et al.: Familial systemic lupus erythematosus in males. Arthritis Rheum 26:39–44, 1983
160. Reinertsen JL, Klippel JH, Johnson AH, et al.: Family studies of B lymphocyte alloantigens in systemic lupus erythematosus. J Rheumatol 9:253–262, 1982
161. Sano H, Imokawa M, Steinberg AD, et al.: Accumulation of guanine-cytosine enriched low M.W.: DNA fragments in lymphocytes of patients with systemic lupus erythematosus. J Immunol 130:187–190, 1983
162. Lahita RG, Bradlow L, Fishman J, et al.: Estrogen metabolism in systemic lupus erythematosus: Patients and family members. Arthritis Rheum 25:843–846, 1982
163. Miller KB, Schwartz RS: Familial abnormalities of suppressor-cell function in systemic lupus erythematosus. N Engl J Med 301:803, 1979
164. Reinertsen JL, Klippel JH, Johnson AH, et al.: B lymphocyte alloantigens associated with systemic lupus erythematosus. N Engl J Med 299:515, 1978
165. Lawley TJ, Hall RP, Fauci AS, et al.: Defective Fc-receptor functions associated with HLA-B8/DR3 haplotype. N Engl J Med 304:185–192, 1982
166. Wilson JG, Wong WW, Schur PH, et al.: Mode of inheritance of decreased C3b receptors on erythrocyte of patients with systemic lupus erythematosus. N Engl J Med 307:981–986, 1982
167. Taurog JD, Moutsopoulos HM, Rosenberg YJ, et al.: The CBA/N X-linked defect prevents NZB B-cell hyperactivity in F_1 mice. J Exp Med 150:31–43, 1979
168. Taurog JD, Raveche ES, Smathers PA, et al.: T cell abnormalities in NZB mice occur independently of autoantibody production. J Exp Med 153:221–234, 1981
169. Steinberg BJ, Smathers PA, Frederiksen K, et al.: Ability of the *xid* gene to prevent autoimmunity in (NZB × NZW) F_1 mice during the course of their natural history, after polyclonal stimulation or following immunization with DNA. J Clin Invest 70:587–597, 1982
170. Smith HR, Chused TM, Steinberg AD: The effect of the X-linked immune deficiency gene *(xid)* upon the Y chromosome related disease of BXSB mice. J Immunol 131:1257–1262, 1983
171. Prickett JD, Robinson DR, Steinberg AD: Dietary enrichment with the polyunsa-

turated fatty acid eicosopentaenoic acid prevents proteinuria and prolongs survival in NZB × NZW F_1 mice. J Clin Invest 68:556–559, 1981

172. Prickett JD, Robinson DR, Steinberg AD: Effects of dietary enrichment with eicosapentanoic acid upon autoimmune nephritis in female (NZB × NZW) F_1 mice. Arthritis Rheum 26:133–139, 1983

Barbara S. Nepom
Jane G. Schaller

2

Childhood Systemic Lupus Erythematosus

Systemic lupus erythematosus (SLE) is a multisystem disease with protean manifestations. Although its causes remain elusive, it is a disease characterized by faulty functioning of the immune system with the formation of numerous aberrant self-reactive antibodies (autoantibodies); much of the tissue injury that causes the clinical manifestations of disease is immunologically mediated in the form of immune complex disease. As the basic causes remain uncertain, so does its optimum treatment. Available treatment modalities have potentially life-threatening side effects, so the physician must strike a balance between the dangers of the disease and the dangers of therapy.

In children with SLE this dilemma is intensified. A number of reports have discussed SLE in children.[1-12] Although the disease itself is predominantly the same in children as in adults, disease course in childhood lupus tends to be acute and severe. Rapid diagnosis and evaluation and aggressive therapy are thus important to disease outcome. On the other hand, aggressive treatment in the growing child can cause serious and even permanent side effects. Careful evaluation and frequent follow-up, therefore, are important. Furthermore, attention must be paid to the child's growth and development and psychosocial needs. Early recognition of complications can allow prompt intervention and can potentially minimize the effects of the disease on the child and family; therefore, knowledge of the myriad possible disease manifestations is necessary.

In this review we will begin with a description of the presenting features of childhood lupus and a summary of factors associated with the disease.

PROGRESS IN CLINICAL RHEUMATOLOGY VOL. I ISBN 0-8089-1646-7

The major portion of the review will then describe the protean manifestations of SLE in children, using an organ–system approach. We will then address appropriate laboratory studies, modes of therapy, and eventual outcome. Lupus phenomena in infants born to mothers with SLE and the entity of "neonatal lupus" will also be discussed.

PRESENTING FEATURES

Symptoms of childhood SLE may begin acutely in a matter of days or insidiously over a long period of time. The most frequent initial manifestations in children include fever, malaise, joint complaints, and rash. A wide variety of findings, however, may be the presenting feature of SLE; these include pleural effusions, pulmonary infiltrates, pericarditis, hemolytic anemia, thrombocytopenia, abdominal pain, seizures, lymphadenopathy, weakness, chest pain, and even recurrent parotid swelling. Most children with SLE have multisystem disease at presentation (Table 2-1).

Criteria for diagnosis of SLE are as necessary in children as in adults. The most recent criteria prepared by the American Rheumatism Association Subcommittee for SLE[13] are listed in Table 2-2.

The diagnosis of SLE in children is usually straightforward. Considerable diagnostic confusion may occur, however, and half of the children in one series has been initially diagnosed as having diseases other than lupus.[4] Rheumatic fever was the most common erroneous initial diagnosis, followed by juvenile rheumatoid arthritis, discoid lupus, sickle cell anemia, Hodgkin's disease, idiopathic thrombocytopenic purpura, and reticuloendotheliosis.

Unlike adults, children rarely have mild lupus; isolated discoid lupus also is unusual. Instead, most children have an acute, severe course with life-threatening manifestations at some time during the disease. It is therefore important to evaluate major system involvement thoroughly at the time of diagnosis and begin treatment promptly. Workup should include, in addition to a careful history and physical exam, complete blood count, platelet count, sedimentation rate, antinuclear antibodies, complement levels (CH50, C_3, C_4), DNA binding, BUN, creatinine, chest x-ray, electrocardiogram, and urinalysis. Electroencephalogram, CAT or brain scan, renal biopsy, pulmonary function tests, GI series, or echocardiography may also be helpful. Initial evaluation should be promptly done so as not to delay proper treatment.

Table 2-1
Clinical Signs and Symptoms Present at the Time of Diagnosis of Childhood SLE
(% of patients)

Reference	Total patients	Arthritis/ arthralgia	Fever	Rash	Alopecia	Nephritis	Lymphadenopathy and/or hepato-splenomegaly	Psychiatric	Serositis	Seizures	Cardio-vascular	CNS	Pulmonary	GI	Hemolytic anemia	Thrombo-phlebitis	Bleeding/ thrombocytopenia	Weight loss	Ophthalmolgic	Edema	Myalgia	Malaise/ fatigue	Oral/nasal ulcers	Photo-sensitivity	Raynaud's	Vasculitis
Meislin and Rothfield[4]	42	88	90	74		52	64	14			31	24	21	14				43				57		31		9
Walravens and Chase[127]	50	84	74	76			44				28	18	40	33			41	36	5	30	47	48	15		5	
Coleman et al.[6]	39	70	92	70	10	52	54				65	10	49					31								
Fish et al.[7]	49	57	63	78			31							18												
King et al.[8]	108	79		70		61	67				17	13	19													
Norris et al.[9]	101	84	68							6		18						31				58				
Wallace et al.[10]	45	64		51	9	63		2		2	24	18	44				20				36		38			
Caeiro et al.[11]	42	38	16	21	2	2			2	2					9	9									2	2

Table 2-2
The 1982 Revised Criteria for Classification of Systemic Lupus Erythematosus*

Malar rash
Discoid rash
Photosensitivity
Oral ulcers
Arthritis of 2 or more joints
Serositis
Pleuritis or
pericarditis
Renal disorder
Persistent proteinuria or
cellular casts
Neurologic disorder
Seizures or
psychosis
Hematologic disorder
Hemolytic anemia or
leukopenia or
lymphopenia or
thrombocytopenia
Immunologic disorder
Positive LE cell preparation or
anti-DNA antibody or
anti-Sm antibody or
false positive serologic test for syphilis
Antinuclear antibody

*The proposed classification is based on 11 criteria. For the purpose of identifying patients in clinical studies, a person shall be said to have systemic lupus erythematosus if any 4 or more of the 11 criteria are present, serially or simultaneously, during any interval of observation.[13]

FACTORS ASSOCIATED WITH SYSTEMIC LUPUS ERYTHEMATOSUS IN CHILDREN

Genetic Associations

The relative importance of genetic and environmental factors in SLE has not been determined, although both have been implicated. Genetic influences are suggested by the greater concordance for SLE in monozygotic as compared to dizygotic twins.[14–16] On the other hand, a higher than expected incidence of lymphocytotoxic antibodies in both consanguineous and nonconsanguineous relatives of SLE patients suggests the possibility of an environmental agent as a factor in disease expression.[17–20]

Familial SLE has long been noted in adults. In one study, Buckman et al. found that 12 percent of 340 lupus patients had affected relatives; 10 percent of the females and 30 percent of the males fell into this group.[21] Statistics in children are similar. King et al.[8] found 15 of 108 children with SLE to have relatives of all ages with the same disease. Another smaller study showed that 12 percent of children with SLE had a family history of connective tissue disease.[6]

Recently, many studies have attempted to link this apparent genetic susceptibility to the HLA loci, the major histocompatibility complex in man. While several investigators have found an association with either HLA-DR2, HLA-DR3, or HLA-B8 (which is in linkage dysequilibrium with DR3),[22–26] extensive studies exclusively in children have not been reported.

Isolated Immune Deficiencies

Children with genetic deficiencies of complement components have an increased risk of developing SLE. Deficiencies of C1, C2, and C4 have been described but are presumably rare.[27–33)] Petty et al,[34] have also reported an association of IgA deficiency and lupus. Diagnosis of lupus in a very young child should raise one's suspicions of these associations.

Drug-Induced SLE

As in adults, drugs have been associated with SLE-like syndromes in children. While hydralazine, procainamide, and isoniazid are common offenders in adults, children are most frequently affected after administration of anticonvulsants, especially hydantoin compounds, trimethadione, and ethosuximide. At least 24 children have been described in the literature with presumed anticonvulsant-induced SLE syndromes.[2,4,35] Fever, arthritis, and rash were the most common presenting symptoms, and other organ involvement included pericarditis, pleural effusions, and renal disease, which led to death in 3 cases. Singsen et al.[35] studied in detail 5 children with ethosuximide-induced disease and found similar manifestations. Symptoms disappeared with the discontinuation of the drug in 4 of 5 children; the other continued to have active lupus nephritis. In these cases, however, it can be difficult to determine whether the drug is truly responsible for inducing the disease or whether the seizure disorder is the initial manifestation of SLE.

Antinuclear antibodies (ANA) among children taking anticonvulsants are more common. Beernink and Miller[36] found a 23 percent incidence of ANA among 48 asymptomatic children taking trimethadione, ethosuximide, or hydantoin, while Singsen et al. found 20 percent with positive ANA's among children receiving either of the latter two drugs.[35] Furthermore, follow-up of 6–12 months revealed that none of the ANA-positive asymptomatic children developed clinical evidence of SLE even though they remained on the same medications; this suggests that a positive ANA alone is not an indication for discontinuation of the anticonvulsant.

Age, Sex, Racial Factors

Comprehensive incidence and prevalence statistics of SLE in children have not been reported. In American adults, the annual incidence has been estimated at about 6–8 cases per 100,000 population,[37] with a prevalence of about 1 in 2000. When broken down into specific subgroups of patients, however, the numbers may be much higher, approaching 1 case per 245 black women in San Francisco and 1 case per 700 women of all races between the ages of 15 and 64 years. Children under the age of 16 years account for about 20 percent of all cases of SLE.[4]

Occasional case reports describe lupus-like syndromes in children as young as 1–2 years of age.[38] Occurrence before the age of 6–8 years, however, is unusual. The incidence rises with increasing age, with the peak age of onset in the 15–25-year age group.[39] The time between onset of symptoms and diagnosis may be quite long, more than 10 years in some reports.[11]

As in adults, female children are affected much more commonly than males, but the ratios of affected females to males are lower in younger patients. In a compilation of several childhood series, Hanson notes an overall total of 80 males and 363 females, 18 and 82 percent, respectively.[40] This contrasts with a 10.9 percent male incidence reported in adults. Further, when divided into groups of patients whose disease begins before or after puberty, the difference in ratios of girls to boys is even more pronounced: 2 or 3 to 1 in the younger group, compared to about 8 in 1 in the postpubertal group.[8,10,12]

The disease can occur in any race. As mentioned above, the incidence of SLE among black women is significantly higher than that among white women. This higher frequency among distinct racial groups seems to hold true with children as well.[8,10] Besides Caucasians and blacks, childhood SLE has also been reported in Hispanics, Orientals, Mexicans, Philippinos, Hawaiians, and native Americans.[8,39]

CLINICAL MANIFESTATIONS

Systemic Symptoms

Nearly all children with SLE have general systemic symptoms, such as fever and fatigue, early in the course of their disease (Table 2-3). Symptoms may begin either acutely or insidiously and occasionally occur years before

Table 2-3
Signs and Symptoms Present Throughout the Course of Childhood SLE

(% of patients)

Reference	Total patients	Malaise	Rash	Hematologic abnormality	Fever	Nephritis	Musculo-skeletal	Pleural/pulmonary	Hepatospleno-megaly or adenopathy	Neuro-psychiatric	Cardiac	Weight loss	Hypertension	Ocular	GI	Raynaud's	Edema	Mucous membrane ulcerations	vasculitis
Meislin and Rothfield[4]	42		79	52		69	90	26	69	62	38				24				
Fish et al.[7]	49					37				28	30								
King et al.[8]	108		44			60	34	13	20	19	17				11				
Norris et al.[9]	101		55				61	10	34	8	9		14	8			28	22	
Wallace et al.[10]	45	96	96	91	84	84	82	67	58	49	42	38	33	31	29	13		49	
Caeiro et al.[11]	42		76		55	48	100	36	41	57	24					31		19	55

the diagnosis of SLE is made. Most children with SLE appear to be systemically ill at the time of diagnosis. Fever in childhood lupus is a common finding.[10,11] It may be intermittent or sustained, low grade or high. The occurrence of fever, however, should always prompt a search for infection; even before steroid treatment is instituted, infection is one of the leading causes of morbidity and mortality in SLE.[39]

Fatigue and malaise are also frequent early complaints in childhood lupus; they occur in up to 96 percent of patients.[10] Weight loss and/or growth retardation are reported in 38 percent in children in the same series. Lymphadenopathy is common, occurring in up to 50 percent of patients.[6,9,11]

Other symptoms frequently that occur early in the disease course include headache, not clearly related to CNS involvement, and sore throat without evidence of infectious origin. Incidence of these symptoms has been reported as 13 percent and 16 percent, respectively.

Cutaneous Abnormalities

Cutaneous lesions are extremely varied in children with SLE but occur in some form in nearly 80 percent of patients; this makes rash one of the most frequent manifestations of SLE. The classic macular or papular erythematous butterfly rash across the cheeks and bridge of the nose is present in about 50 percent of affected children and may occur early or late in disease course. This rash may be precipitated by sun exposure. Usually this rash heals well with treatment and leaves no scars. Typical discoid lesions may also occur in the course of systemic disease.

Macular lesions on the hands, feet, and trunk are also quite common in children; they occur in about 25 percent of patients. Other rashes can be noted in widely varying patterns: purpura, bullae, ulcerating lesions, recurrent hives, and nodules have all been described.[40–44] Even lupus panniculitis has recently been reported in a child.[45]

Mucocutaneous lesions are also quite common; they occur in up to 50 percent of patients.[41] Erythematous or bullous lesions of the hard palate were present in 21 percent of children at disease onset in one series[8]; oral ulcers were seen in 19 percent of children in another study.[11]

The study by Caeiro et al.[11] of 42 children with SLE, vasculitis (digital vasculitis, nail-fold infarcts, palmar and plantar rashes, or skin ulcerations) was present in 55 percent of patients, purpura in 17 percent (half not associated with thrombocytopenia), discoid lesions in 7 percent, and small rheumatoid-like nodules on the elbow developed in one patient.

Alopecia, either patchy or generalized, occurs in up to 50 percent of children; this may be present early, especially in children with rash. The hair will regrow normally with treatment of the systemic illness, unless the underlying scalp lesion is a discoid lesion, in which case the hair loss may be permanent.

Raynaud's phenomenon has been reported in up to 33 percent of children.[10,11] Photosensitivity occurs in about 30 percent of children[11] and may vary widely in severity; this occasionally precipitates severe urticaria, bullous lesions, or even systemic disease.[39] It is unusual for photosensitivity to begin after the first year or so of disease.

Hematologic Abnormalities

Hematologic abnormalities are also common in childhood.[46] Nearly every patient will manifest at least one of these features at some time during disease duration; many of these occur at presentation or early in disease course. Although usually treatment aimed at the underlying disease improves hematologic parameters as well, these abnormalities may occasionally be life threatening.

Anemia is probably the most common hematologic abnormality, with an incidence variously reported as 52, 66, and 80 percent of children.[6,9,11] The most common basis of this anemia is not, in fact, autoimmune in nature, but is the "anemia of chronic disease," with normocytic normochromic indices, normal bone marrow appearance, and adequate marrow iron stores.[46] Serum iron and total iron-binding capacity may be reduced, but there is no response to treatment with iron. When iron-deficiency anemia is occasionally present in lupus patients, it is usually secondary to gastrointestinal losses.

Hemolytic anemia on an immune basis may also occur in childhood lupus but has been reported in only 3–10 percent of cases.[9,11] Up to 33 percent of children may have positive Coombs' tests, however.[10,46] Antierythrocyte antibodies are often IgGs of the "warm" variety[46]; cold agglutinins associated with hemolytic anemia in lupus are rare. A recent case report has described an 11-year-old girl who displayed an autoerythrocyte sensitization syndrome as the primary manifestation of SLE; this is the only instance reported in a child.[47]

Leukopenia is another very common abnormality in children with SLE; it occurs in over 50 percent of patients.[46] These patients may have a decrease in the number of circulating lymphocytes, or granulocytes, or both. Absolute levels of peripheral granulocytes may be strikingly decreased. While antigranulocyte antibodies have been proposed as a mechanism for this decrease, the evidence is not yet convincing. In addition, some authors have suggested the possibility of central bone marrow suppression of granulopoiesis in lupus but, again, this requires confirmation. Finally, increased adhesiveness of neutrophils may help account for observed neutropenia.[48]

Lymphopenia is quite often present in periods of active disease. Both the absolute levels of lymphocytes and their relative percentages may be reduced when compared to other cell types. Rivero et al.,[49] in a study of 158 untreated patients of all ages with active SLE, found that 93 percent of patients had lymphopenia at some time during the course of their disease, that lymphopenia occurred more frequently than any other criteria for classification of SLE, and that it was the most common initial laboratory abnormality. The existence of circulating cytotoxic antilymphocyte antibody in SLE has been well established.[50–52] These antibodies are usually active at reduced temperatures, require complement, and have been correlated with lower leukocyte and C3 levels as well as with increased hematologic and other organ system symptomatology.

Thrombocytopenia affects about 33% of children with SLE[46]; occasionally this abnormality may precede other evidence of lupus, and these children are initially diagnosed as having idiopathic thrombocytopenic purpura. Patients may show shortened platelet survival time, with increased numbers of megakaryocytes seen in the bone marrow. This may occur as a compensated state, with resultant normal counts of circulating platelets. Platelets from lupus patients may fix complement without the addition of exogenous serum, which implies the presence of antibody of immune complexes on their surfaces.[46] It is thought that platelet destruction in these cases is primarily mediated by IgG antibodies, but recent studies have shown some patients to have immune thrombocytopenia without increased levels of platelet-associated IgG; this suggests that another class of antibody may also be involved.

Again, steroid therapy will usually improve this condition, but splenectomy may be needed in refractory cases. In these situations, pathology of the spleen may be helpful if the diagnosis is still uncertain, since the characteristic periarterial concentric fibrosis often seen in lupus (onion-skin lesion) is not present in truly idiopathic thrombocytopenic purpura.

Circulating anticoagulants occur in at least 25 percent of children with SLE and may cause clinically significant bleeding.[46] The presence of these anticoagulants is strongly associated with a chronic false-positive reaction for syphilis, and both measures may appear and disappear together, according to disease.[39,53] These anticoagulants are directed against many of the clotting components, including factors XI, IX, VIII, prothrombin, antithrombin, and the phospholipid component of the prothrombin activator complex.[53,54] These anticoagulant effects, although not usually causing significant spontaneous bleeding, may become important when invasive procedures, such as renal biopsy, are considered. Most of these effects are reversible with corticosteroids.

While most children with SLE at some time express one or more of these hematologic abnormalities, it has been suggested that some of these dysfunctions may represent specific subsets of lupus, with different prognoses and therapeutic requirements. Alger et al.[55] studied 31 lupus patients with hemolytic anemia and/or thrombocytopenic purpura and found these patients to be significantly younger, more often male, and with less frequent systemic manifestations of disease; they also appear to have a more benign overall disease course. If these subsets hold up in other investigations, they may be a useful way of separating a distinct group of patients.

Renal Involvement

Renal involvement in children with SLE, as in adults, has been responsible for much of the morbidity and mortality of the disease. At least 80 percent of children with SLE demonstrate clinical or laboratory evidence of renal involvement (abnormal urinalysis, hypertension, renal insufficiency),[10] with a range of 44–88 percent.[11,56] Usually, renal involvement is present early in the course of disease but can develop many years after diagnosis of SLE.

Pathologic classification of renal disease is the same as that used in adults.[57–60] Mesangial, or minimal, nephritis is characterized by immunoglobulin and often C3 deposits in mesangial regions, with or without mild mesangial proliferation visible on light microscopy, with mesangial deposits by electron microscopy (EM). Membranous nephropathy shows diffuse capillary wall thickening, immunoglobulin, and C3 deposits in capillary walls, and subepithelial deposits along basement membranes by EM. Focal glomerulonephritis has mesangial endothelial proliferation and some capillary wall thickening, described as the "wire-loop" lesion, as well as leukocyte infiltration; these abnormalities are seen only in certain segments of glomeruli while over 50 percent appear normal by light microscopy. On EM, there are electron dense deposits, they are primarily found in the mesangium but also occasionally are found in the subendothelial space. Immunofluorescence shows focal mesangial deposits of immunoglobulins or complement components. The last type is designated "diffuse proliferative glomerulonephritis" and is the most common lesion in children. These defects are similar to the focal glomerulonephritis type but are much more extensive; they involve over 90 percent of glomeruli. The mesangial matrix is markedly increased. Immunoglobulin deposits are more abundant, and electron dense deposits are more generalized; they occur in the subendothelial, mesangial, and subepithelial areas.[58–59]

Beyond these four basic histological types, another pattern may be rarely associated with lupus in children. Libit et al.[61] described the distinctive pathologic changes in childhood extramembranous glomerulonephritis, an uncommon lesion that is often associated with nephrotic syndrome. In their small study, they describe 7 children with this entity, 3 of whom went on to develop SLE. They conclude that children with the diagnosis of extramembranous glomerulonephritis demand close, careful follow-up for future evidence of SLE.

The most common histologic lesion of those children who undergo renal biopsy for lupus is diffuse proliferative glomerulonephritis. Frequency of this type of renal history in children has been variously reported from 30 to 70 percent.[7,8,12,60,62] The frequency of the other types varies considerably among authors, with all three types ranging from about 5 to 35 percent.

In adults, progression from one histologic type of lesion to another has been well described, although uncommon. The same appears to be true in children. In the report of Mahajan et al. of 41 SLE patients of all ages who had repeat renal biopsies 3 months to 5 years after their first biopsies, 66 percent of patients with focal glomerulonephritis progressed to diffuse glomerulonephritis (7 patients) or membranous nephropathy (3 patients); changes in histologic pattern of the other types was uncommon.[63] Of those 41 patients, only 1 showed improvement on repeat biopsy. In the study of Morris et al. of children, 2 of only 4 patients rebiopsied showed worsening of the histologic picture.[57] Cassidy et al.[56] describe one girl who developed diffuse proliferative glomerulonephritis 4 years after a biopsy that showed focal glomerulonephritis. The study by Garin et al.[62] also reports 2 children whose repeat renal biopsy showed diffuse proliferative glomerulonephritis, whereas the initial histology had been focal proliferative glomerulonephritis. In addition, he describes 3 other patients whose renal biopsies improved. Further studies are necessary to determine the true incidence of changing renal biopsy in childhood SLE.

Morris et al.[57] also studied the mode of presentation of renal disease in children with SLE and related it to the renal biopsy results. He found that, although all 36 of his patients had evidence of nephritis at some time during the course of their disease, few had significant renal disease at presentation. Of those with early renal disease, presentation included the nephrotic syndrome and persistent proteinuria.

Correlation of histologic renal disease is imperfect. In general, diffuse proliferative glomerulonephritis is accompanied by abnormal urinalyses, with hematuria, RBC casts, or proteinuria; this sometimes leads to the nephrotic syndrome. Renal insufficiency and hypertension may occur. From a different perspective, 21 of 22 SLE patients who presented with nephrotic syndrome displayed proliferative glomerulonephritis on biopsy.[57] Patients with focal glomerulonephritis, on the other hand, rarely develop nephrotic syndrome or renal failure. Clinically their renal disease is usually restricted to microscopic proteinuria and hematuria. Those with membranous nephropathy frequently develop the nephrotic syndrome and occasionally go on to renal failure and/or hypertension. Minimal nephritis has the fewest clinical manifestations; it usually shows only microscopic urinary abnormalities but can occasionally progress to nephrotic syndrome or renal failure.

Renal biopsy has been felt to be an important predictor of outcome in lupus, although it is not infallible. In fact, one recent report of SLE in adults concluded there was no difference in long-term outcome of the different histological groups.[64] Most authors, however, suggest that the diffuse proliferative group has the worst prognosis. In our series[10] 50 percent of children with diffuse proliferative glomerulonephritis had clinically normal renal status at median disease duration. Garin et al. estimated a 5-year survival rate of only 60.9 percent in their group of children with diffuse proliferative glomerulonephritis,[62] while Fish et al.[7] report a 73 percent 10-year survival rate for that group and an 87 percent rate for children with focal glomerulonephritis. Prediction of which children will do well and which will pursue a downhill course is still uncertain, even with renal biopsy data. One intriguing point was made by Comerford and Cohen,[65] who suggested that the most important feature characterizing adult lupus patients with a favorable outcome was the complete disappearance of subendothelial deposits on renal biopsies repeated 1–2 years after the onset of therapy. Whether this holds up in future studies of children remains to be seen.

Several recent studies have focused on the discrepancy between lupus nephropathy and clinical renal involvement, the so-called "occult" or "silent" renal disease. It had been known for some time that lupus patients with extrarenal manifestations but without clinical renal features could have abnormal renal biopsies, but these were usually felt to occur in the "minimal change" histologic group. Mahajan et al.,[66] however, studied the renal biopsies of 27 adults with SLE and no clinical renal dysfunction and found, surprisingly, that 12 of them had diffuse proliferative glomerulonephritis, most with moderate to marked inflammatory activity. Subsequently, Woolf and his colleagues[67] identified 8 children with SLE and normal renal function as evaluated by urinalysis, creatinine clearance, and 24-hour urine protein measurement. On renal biopsy, 3 patients had generalized segmental, 2 had focal segmental, and 1 had diffuse proliferative glomerulonephritis. Furthermore, all 8 children were found to have immune complex deposition shown by immunofluorescence or electron microscopy. Similarly, Weis et al. obtained renal biopsies from 4 adolescent girls with symptomatic thrombocytopenia, serologic evidence of SLE, and no clinical signs of renal involvement.[68] All 4 showed varying degrees of glomerular disease by immunofluorescence or electron microscopic studies, although only 2 were abnormal by light microscopy. Repeat biopsies later in the course of disease ranged from apparent resolution to significant progression of glomerular disease, highlighting the variable patterns of occult lupus glomerulonephritis.

Thus, it appears that even among childhood SLE patients with clinically normal renal function and normal urinalysis, the kidneys may be significantly involved. This underlines the dilemma of when to obtain a renal biopsy, since one might be more aggressive therapeutically knowing the kidneys were actively involved. Until large series are reported, however, the question remains unanswered.

Musculoskeletal Involvement

Joint involvement is one of the most common early manifestations of SLE. In one series,[39] arthritis was present in 78 percent of patients of all ages at the time of diagnosis, and 86 percent developed arthritis at some time during the disease course. Incidence in childhood is similarly high: Caeiro et al.[11] found 100 percent of children had arthritis or arthralgias, and in 38 percent it was presenting complaint. Norris et al. found nondeforming arthritis in over 60 percent of children with SLE,[9] while Coleman et al.'s study found 70 percent with joint complaints.[6]

The arthritis in children, as in adults, is characteristically nondeforming and nonerosive, although Jaccoud's deforming arthritis (JRA) was described in 4 of 42 childhood lupus patients in one study.[11] More typically, multiple large joints are involved, such as the knees, hips, shoulders, and elbows, usually in a migratory pattern. Rarely the disease may present as a monarthritis, and at times the chronicity of symptoms may confuse the diagnosis with that of JRA. Ragsdale et al.[69] describe 10 patients initially diagnosed as JRA who went on to develop obvious clinical manifestations of SLE 2–21 years later. Another disease occasionally confused with early SLE in children because of the nature of the arthritis is rheumatic fever. Usually, however, enough other systems are involved in lupus that the diagnosis is clear. Periostitis may also lead to musculoskeletal complaints in SLE.

Muscle involvement can also occur. In adult series, incidence of myositis is about 5–10 percent.[70,71] Childhood series include a frequency of myalgia of 47 percent in one study,[6] and proximal muscle weakness in 14 percent in another report.[11] Many investigators do not list myositis separately, however, and large-scale studies of children that include muscle biopsies are lacking. Study of lupus myositis is further complicated by the possible occurrence of myositis as a result of either corticosteroid or antimalarial drug therapy. It seems clear, however, that true lupus myopathy unrelated to treatment can occur; it is often mild, characterized by pain, tenderness, weakness (often in a proximal distribution), and elevated serum levels of muscle enzymes. Tsokos et al. found the serum aldolase level to be much more helpful than the creatinine phosphokinase in this situation.[70]

Another complication among patients with SLE is avascular necrosis, described by Dubois and Cozen in 1960.[72] Although initially reported in adults, it has become clear that younger patients also can develop this entity, perhaps even with a greater incidence than adults. While the reported incidence of avascular necrosis in adult series is approximately 5–12 percent,[73,74] in children it approaches 40 percent. Hurley et al.[75] describe symptomatic avascular necrosis of the femoral head in 4 of 10 children followed for SLE. They note the insidious nature of the symptoms, which often predate the radiologic diagnosis by weeks or months, although usually symptoms occur late in disease course. Bergstein et al.[76] performed skeletal radiological surveys on 35 children with SLE to determine the prevalence of avascular necrosis. Fourteen patients, or 40 percent, had avascular necrosis of a total of 31 bones. The most common sites included, in descending order of frequency, the femoral condyle, femoral head, talus, capitulum of elbow, metatarsals, and patella. No significant differences were found between those with and those without avascular necrosis in terms of age at onset of SLE, duration of prednisone or azathioprine therapy, or the average prednisone dose.

Although most investigators agree that the most common sites of avascular necrosis are weight-bearing joints, one study describes the involvement of the wrist in this process.[77] Again, the onset of pain was insidious and in most cases the symptoms were thought to be due to lupus synovitis; this leads to an average 11-month delay between the onset of symptoms and the diagnosis.

The cause of avascular necrosis remains unclear. Corticosteroid administration is a presumed major contributor to the process, since avascular necrosis is also seen frequently in many non-SLE syndromes treated with steroids, such as nephrotic syndrome, hematologic disorders, rheumatoid arthritis, and renal transplantation. Most SLE studies cannot define a significant association between incidence of avascular necrosis and duration of dosage of steroid therapy, however. Furthermore, a small number of untreated SLE patients have also developed avascular necrosis; this led some to speculate that the underlying disease and the treatment may each be etiologically involved.[78,79]

Whatever the underlying pathogenesis, clearly avascular necrosis is not an uncommon complication in childhood lupus. Diagnosis may be difficult because of insidious onset of symptoms, the similarity of symptoms to those of lupus synovitis, the presence of asymptomatic cases, and the delay between onset of avascular necrosis and radiographic changes. In addition, avascular necrosis may become apparent in patients who are entering a quiescent or relatively inactive phase of their lupus, possibly due to an increase in physical activity that precipitates articular collapse.[80] Broader awareness of this complication, which can have significant sequelae, particularly in the growing child, will lead to more prompt and accurate diagnosis and appropriate therapy.

Cardiovascular Involvement

Approximately 30 to 40 percent of children with SLE will at some time develop cardiac involvement from their disease.[4,7,11] The most common of these is pericarditis; it occurs in 23.8 percent of cases in one childhood study.[11] Pericardial thickening alone, without effusions, may be detected by echocardiography. One report found thickening in 41 percent of patients studied prospectively.[81] The one patient who died during the study showed adhesive pericarditis at autopsy. Pericarditis occurs with pericardial effusions in up to 25 percent of cases. In a Japanese study of adults[82] with SLE, 53 percent of patients with active disease had pericardial effusions as detected by cardiac echo. Other studies have found much lower frequencies, probably due to different detection methods, but many authors agree that the incidence seems to be somewhat lower in younger patients.[83]

Symptoms include pleuritic or substernal pain, but pericarditis may present primarily as dyspnea or as a cardiac arrhythmia. Chest x-ray may reveal an enlarged cardiac shadow, but the heart is rarely massively enlarged. EKG shows T-wave abnormalities. Tamponade is the most frequent and serious complication, which occurs in approximately 7 percent of cases of SLE pericarditis.[83] Constrictive pericarditis, on the other hand, is exceedingly rare, reported in only a few patients. It can occur in younger patients, however, as described by Jacobson and Reza in a case report of a 17-year-old male who presented with clinical signs of severe constrictive pericarditis.[84] Surgery, which removed the fibrous pericardium, was curative. Interestingly, immunopathology of the tissue showed IgG, IgM, and C3 deposition on its surface, which implies an immunological basis to this rare complication.

The classic endocardial lesions of lupus, Libman–Sacks endocarditis, rarely cause clinically significant pathology, although new cardiac murmurs may be noted. It is not uncommon to observe these changes at necropsy, however. Irregular thickening of valve leaflets or more obvious vegetations may be seen on echocardiogram, but rarely are these hemodynamically significant. A single case has been reported where Libman–Sacks endocarditis caused progressive, life-threatening mitral regurgitation in an 18-year-old male, which required mitral valve replacement.[85]

Myocardial infarction and ischemia have more recently been recognized as complications of lupus, even in the younger patient. Perhaps the most striking example is a case of sudden death from myocardial infarction in a 5-year-old child with SLE.[86] It is postulated that in her case, coronary artery atherosclerosis may have been accelerated by hypertriglyceridemia and prolonged steroid therapy superimposed on a hypersensitivity vasculitis associated with her underlying lupus. Meller et al.[87] describe 3 young adults with SLE who had infarctions. Two had electrocardiographic changes consistent with infarction but without symptoms. The third developed fatal acute myocardial infarction with cardiogenic shock. Six further cases of ischemic heart disease in young adults with SLE have recently been reported.[88] Of these, two showed coronary arteritis and two showed coronary atherosclerosis at autopsy; another had abnormal coronary angiography, which later improved after the institution of steroids; the final patient eventually underwent coronary bypass surgery for relief of angina. The authors conclude that, although rare, coronary artery disease can occur in association with lupus, sometimes in the absence of extracardiac manifestations. Steroid therapy and angiography should be considered when this is suspected. Finally, a report of necropsy patients studied the frequency and severity of coronary artery narrowing in 22 young adults with SLE.[89] Nearly 50 percent of those studied had severe narrowing of at least one of the four major coronary arteries. The existence of this severe narrowing correlated with increased serum cholesterol increased mean systolic/diastolic systemic arterial pressures, increased frequency of mitral valve disease, and increased frequency of pericardial adhesions.

Myocarditis may occur as part of SLE as well, heralded either by poor cardiac function, cardiomegaly, or conduction defects. One study of cardiac function by noninvasive means disclosed evidence of left ventricular dysfunction, even in the younger patients, which could not be attributed to factors such as age, duration of disease, renal involvement, hypertension, steroid treatment, or immunological activity.[90] Conduction defects are another manifestation presumably due to myocardial involvement near the sinoatrial (SA) or atrioventricular (AV) nodes. Unusual, serious arrhythmias can occur in younger patients. Bharati et al.[91] describe a 12-year-old girl with SLE where complete AV block was the terminal event; at autopsy, both the SA and AV nodes were nearly completely replaced by granulation tissue. Another group reports a patient with SLE diagnosed at age 18 years of age who developed slowly progressive EKG changes over a 16-year period, which eventually led to complete AV block and required a pacemaker.[92]

Interestingly, many of these cardiac abnormalities can occur simultaneously, which suggests an immunologic basis for these lesions. This is further implied by an immunopathologic study of 10 patients at autopsy in whom immune deposits were found frequently in myocardial vessels, the pericardium, valvular stroma, and even around epicardial nerve fibers (in 2 patients).[93]

Pulmonary Disease

The spectrum of pulmonary disease attributed to SLE is broad; it includes pleuritis, pleural effusions, interstitial pneumonitis, interstitial fibrosis, spontaneous pneumothorax, patchy alveolar infiltrates, acute alveolitis, cavitating nodules, edema, and pulmonary hypertension.[94–98] Some of these manifestations may be secondary effects of infection, renal disease, congestive heart failure, etc., rather than directly caused by the SLE; however, clearly the lung can be a primary target in rheumatic disease. Pulmonary involvement can occasionally be a major clinical problem in SLE, and recent studies have found that the lung is rarely spared completely.[95,98] Indeed, up to 88 percent of random SLE patients may have abnormalities on pulmonary function tests,[94] and Fayemi found histopathologic abnormalities in nearly 75 percent of autopsy cases.[96] Interestingly, many patients had no respiratory symptoms or radiological abnormalities. Pulmonary function tests appear to be the most sensitive indicators of lung involvement in SLE; they show most often a pattern of restrictive lung disease or decreased diffusing capacity.[94,97]

Pleuritis or pleural effusions are the most common pulmonary manifestations of SLE in children; they occurred in approximately 30 percent of cases in one study.[11] While most often present at the time of diagnosis of SLE, pleural involvement may occur later in the course of disease. Although pleural effusions are usually bilateral, we have recently reported a 12-year-old girl who presented with unilateral pleural effusion.[99] It has been suggested that evaluation of pleural fluid for immune complexes, LE cells, and complement determinations, as well as for standard measurements of protein, glucose, WBC, etc., may assist in diagnosis when the pleural effusion is a presenting complaint.[100,101] Regardless of clinical picture or diagnosis, however, infection must be absolutely ruled out in each case. Noninfectious pleural effusions in lupus usually respond rapidly to corticosteroid treatment.

A less frequent pulmonary manifestation of lupus in children is a pattern of steroid-responsive diffuse pulmonary infiltrates,[5,11] which can be difficult to distinguish radiologically from viral pneumonia. Other pulmonary infiltrates, which progress to fibrosis, may not respond to steroids; these, too, can be difficult to distinguish from bacterial, viral, or fungal infections.

Finally, a rare but potentially fatal complication of pulmonary involvement is acute pulmonary hemorrhage.[102,103] In most cases, respiratory symptoms of dyspnea, cough, hemoptysis, or chest pain precede the hemorrhage, but in some cases the onset is sudden and unexpected. One report describes a 7-year-old boy with lupus who presented with epistaxis and massive hemoptysis, which required endotracheal intubation, PEEP, platelet transfusion, and high-dose corticosteroids.[104] Other authors have reported a high mortality rate among both adults and children with lupus and pulmonary hemorrhage. One series of 108 children found 7 with episodes of pulmonary hemorrhage; in 4 of those it was the major factor that led to death.[8]

Overall, then, pulmonary involvement may be a troublesome problem in childhood SLE, with pleural effusions and pleuritis being relatively common. Pulmonary function testing is the most sensitive parameter of lung involvement and might reveal a surprisingly high percentage of affected children if performed routinely in a large series. Lung involvement does not seem to correlate with serologic or immunologic factors or with other organ system involvement.[94] It is imperative to rule out infection as a cause of pulmonary changes; biopsy may even be required. Finally, although rare, acute pulmonary hemorrhage is a potentially treatable cause of death; only a high index of suspicion and early, aggressive treatment can ensure survival in these cases.

Central Nervous System Involvement

Involvement of the central nervous system (CNS) in childhood lupus is common, although incidence varies between 9 and 49 percent in reported studies.[4,7,56,10,105] Yancey et al.[105] recently reported a 43 percent incidence of CNS involvement in a series of 37 children with SLE. Interestingly, 81 percent of those involved had CNS complaints at the onset of their SLE. In contrast, an earlier report[4] describes a 25 percent incidence of neurological complaints and a 17 percent incidence of psychiatric problems at the onset of SLE; they found CNS involvement to be the only prominent organ system whose involvement would frequently develop after treatment commenced, even though not present at the time of diagnosis. Cassidy et al.[56] agree that the CNS is the single major organ system whose involvement was often delayed. In their review of 58 children, they found evidence of CNS involvement of 9 percent at the time of diagnosis; it increased to 31 percent as disease progressed. Cerebrospinal fluid (CSF) analysis, electroencephalogram, and CAT scan may all be useful in evaluating CNS involvement.

CNS involvement in childhood lupus displays a wide spectrum of clinical manifestations, usually similar to those seen in adults. Seizure disorders, usually grand mal but also focal motor in type, are one of the most common neurologic signs and, in fact, may be the first manifestation of SLE. As mentioned above, however, when seizures predate the diagnosis of SLE, it may be difficult to distinguish between an anticonvulsant-induced SLE syndrome and the existence of seizures as the first manifestation of SLE. Withdrawal of the anticonvulsant in question may cause disappearance of the lupus syndrome, which will distinguish between the two.[106]

Chorea has been noted to be associated with lupus for some time and can exist months to years before SLE is diagnosed.[107,108] Herd et al.[109] have recently suggested that chorea may occur relatively more frequently in children with SLE than in adults, particularly when it is the presenting symptom of their lupus. Likewise, standard treatment of chorea with haloperidol may be ineffective until the SLE is recognized and treated.

Persistent headache was a frequent symptom in these studies but one that is often difficult to evaluate. The persistence of headache in children with SLE for more than 1 week with no other etiology found should suggest the possibility of CNS lupus.[105]

Cranial nerve palsies are occasionally noted in children, with ophthalmoplegia the most frequent manifestation. Rare patients develop peripheral neuropathies, such as Guillain–Barré syndrome. Other infrequent neurologic signs include optic atrophy, papilledema, ataxia, nystagmus, paraparesis, parkinsonian-like symptoms, aseptic meningitis, and strokes.[4,105,110,111]

Psychiatric disturbances may be a prominent feature of childhood SLE. As in adults, a wide range of symptoms has been described; these include acute organic brain syndrome, psychosis, hallucinations, abnormal short-term memory, depression, slowed mentation, and phobias.[11,105] Incidence in children during the course of their lupus approaches 25 percent, with severe psychoneuroses the most common diagnosis. Again, psychiatric involvement may be difficult to assess, and the differential diagnosis must include steroid side effects, situational depressions, and preexisting disorders unrelated to SLE.

Prognosis of CNS involvement with lupus has been considered in the past to be poor, although a study by Dubois et al.[112] in adults reported that deaths due to CNS disease declined from 26 percent in the years 1950–1955 to only 8 percent in the period 1963–1973. CNS disease has not been listed as a major cause of death in the pediatric literature, however, and in fact several authors list surprisingly few permanent residua from neurologic involvement. For example, Yancey et al.'s study[105] of 16 children with CNS lupus reports 3 children with continuing seizure disorders and 2 with residual psychiatric disorders. They also describe the nearly complete recovery of a 16-year-old girl who developed parkinsonian symptoms and eventually coma, which lasted 2 months. Other authors describe recovery from severe acute cerebrovascular accidents, psychotic episodes, and seizure disorders.[7,106] This improved outlook is due presumably to more recent usage of high-dose corticosteroids as well as cytotoxic agents, but larger-scale definitive studies remain to be done.

In summary, the incidence and manifestations of CNS lupus in children are similar to those seen in adults, although certain features such as chorea may be more common in younger patients. The prognosis may be better than previously believed, and there are many encouraging examples of severe neuropsychiatric disease where resolution with appropriate therapy is nearly complete. CNS involvement, however, remains a serious aspect of childhood SLE.

Gastrointestinal Manifestations

Gastrointestinal (GI) manifestations of childhood lupus can be surprisingly common, although often vague symptoms and concurrent illnesses or drug administration make diagnosis difficult. Abdominal pain occurred in approximately 10 percent of children at the time of diagnosis of lupus in one study, with symptoms of anorexia, nausea, or vomiting present in another 21 percent.[4] In one adult series, 50 percent of patients complained of at least one of these symptoms or of diarrhea.[113] Interestingly, abdominal pain proved to be more common in children than in adults with SLE. The pain is frequently crampy and intermittent, with nonlocalized tenderness on physical examination; it tends to remit with steroid therapy aimed at other manifestations of lupus. The true incidence is difficult to ascertain, since many series do not include the GI system in their studies. Recent descriptions of various aspects of GI involvement, however, suggest that they may be more frequent than previously believed.[113–115]

Vasculitis is believed to be the underlying pathogenesis for much of the gastrointestinal symptomatology in SLE. Indeed, Ropes[116] found evidence of previous peritoneal inflammation in 63 percent of her adult patients studied at autopsy. No similar statistics are available from younger patients for comparison. Acute, nonsurgical peritonitis and ascites secondary to SLE have also been reported; again, incidence in childhood is unknown.

Mesenteric vasculitis is a well-known cause of abdominal pain in SLE and often responds to treatment of the underlying lupus. Intestinal ischemia, which occasionally leads to infarction and even perforation, can be a life-threatening complication, however. Several authors note that, although surgery may be approached with reluctance in a patient with severe, active SLE, the only patients surviving intestinal perforation were those treated with early, aggressive surgical intervention.[39,113] A less-common complication of mesenteric vasculitis is intussusception, reported by Hermann in 1967 in a 5-year-old child.[117] Yet another rare complication is described by Binstadt and L'Heureux in a 15-year-old female with SLE.[118] During a multisystem flare of her lupus, she developed intermittent abdominal pain, diarrhea, and vomiting; at laparotomy, pneumatosis cystoides intestinalis (cystic air collections in bowel submucosal or subserosal layers) with secondary pneumoperitoneum was found, without evidence of bowel perforation.

GI hemorrhage, although not prominently described in children, occurs in about 5 percent of adult lupus patients.[113] Again, multiple etiologies may exist, which include bleeding secondary to ischemic bowel disease, aspirin or other drug usage, coagulopathy, uremia, and stress. Rare cases have been reported in which GI bleeding has been the cause of death.[119]

Protein-losing enteropathy has been described in only a few patients with SLE, one of them a 12-year-old boy.[120] All improved with corticosteroid therapy.

Disturbances of esophageal motility occur with lupus in 10–32 percent of cases.[39,113,121] Symptoms may include dysphagia and regurgitation; radiological studies may be normal or reveal decreased peristalsis, dilatation of the lower esophagus, or esophageal ulcerations.

Pancreatitis has been mentioned infrequently as a manifestation of SLE, but a recent review suggests that it is more common that originally thought and certainly can occur in the younger patient.[114] Of 63 lupus patients who had had serum amylase determinations, most during an episode of abdominal pain, nearly 50 percent had elevated levels. Many authors have ascribed the incidence of hyperamylasemia and pancreatitis in SLE to the use of steroids, but careful statistical comparisons suggest that pancreatitis occurs more frequently in lupus than in other conditions treated with steroids; indeed, there exist several examples of pancreatitis that occur in lupus patients prior to the institution of corticosteroids. In several cases, treatment with steroids led to normalization of serum amylase levels and abrogation of symptoms. Typically, pancreatitis occurs in the setting of multisystem involvement of lupus. In Reynolds' retrospective study of 26 lupus patients with hyperamylasemia, only two complications occurred; a pseudocyst and a pleural effusion.[114] Both responded to steroid therapy. It thus appears that pancreatitis and hyperamylasemia may occur in lupus more frequently than previously thought; in most cases, this is not a serious problem and may in fact be asymptomatic. Corticosteroids have been considered as both a cause and a treatment for pancreatitis in this setting; more thorough prospective studies are needed.

Severe liver disease is uncommon in childhood SLE, although at least one death (in an 8-year-old child with lupus) was attributed to hepatic insufficiency, with massive fatty infiltration of the liver noted histologically.[39] Some hepatic involvement, especially at the onset of lupus, is much more common, however. Hepatomegaly occurs in some 30 percent of younger patients and appears to be more frequent in children than in adults. Elevations of "liver enzymes" are quite common, even in the absence of aspirin or other drug ingestion. Bilirubin levels may also be mildly elevated. Often these laboratory abnormalities revert to normal once the other clinical manifestations of lupus are brought under control. Jaundice in children with lupus is quite uncommon; it occurs in only 2 percent of patients.

One recent review of liver disease in SLE patients of all ages, however, found that hepatic involvement was more frequent than previously thought, with over 50 percent of the 206 patients having at least one abnormal laboratory result; this indicated liver involvement.[115] Twenty-one percent of these patients "met strict criteria for the existence of disease," and 3 eventually died of liver failure. Again, the incidence and severity of hepatic involvement in childhood lupus remains to be clarified.

Overall, then, GI involvement is not a prominent cause of morbidity and mortality in childhood SLE, but increasing recognition of its potential manifestations may lead to more accurate diagnosis when it does occur. Nonlupus-related causes, like chronic active hepatitis, must be ruled out. Both hepatomegaly and abdominal pain appear to be more frequent in children with SLE than in adults. While in most cases these features resolve with treatment directed at the underlying lupus, rare life-threatening complications such as intestinal perforation can occur and require early intervention.

Ophthalmological Manifestations

The true incidence of ophthalmologic manifestations of SLE is unknown; most patients are not routinely evaluated by ophthalmologic exam. In children it appears to be unusual, with 2 of 39 patients in one study[6] and 8 of 101 in another study[9] showing signs of eye involvement. These included cotton-wool exudates (cytoid bodies), hemorrhages, chorioretinitis, cataracts, diplopia, and papilledema.

Ocular involvement can be separated into that apparently due to the SLE itself and that due to drug side effects.[122] The latter are more common, with cataracts induced by corticosteroids the most frequently seen lesion. Usually this occurs in patients treated with high doses of steroids for more than 1 year. Similarly, the retinopathy induced by antimalarials is related to dose and duration of treatment and can lead to irreversible loss of vision.

A wide variety of eye manifestations due to the lupus itself may occur; some of these are secondary to hypertension, vasculitis, or hematologic abnormalities. Included are conjunctivitis, subconjunctival or retinal hemorrhage, episcleritis and scleritis, iridocyclitis, chorioretinitis, and the classic cytoid bodies. Again, these are relatively uncommon in childhood.

Endocrine Disease

Although not commonly recognized in pediatric lupus patients, concomitant symptomatic thyroid disease may occur. While circulating antithyroid antibodies have been described in some patients with SLE, their frequency is not known; usually they occur in euthyroid patients. Richards et al.[123] describe, however, 2 children who developed symptomatic hypothyroidism before or during the course of their lupus. While it is possible that this represents two separate diseases, the presence of antithyroid antibodies in both patients suggests an immune basis for their hypothyroidism. They conclude that this diagnosis be considered in a child with SLE who shows evidence of growth failure, delay of puberty, edema, unexplained pallor, or palpable thyroid gland.

Amenorrhea is also common in lupus patients, as it is with many chronic diseases. In our series, 8 of 34 girls developed this problem.[10]

LABORATORY STUDIES

In general, the characteristic laboratory values for children with SLE are similar to those of adult lupus patients. ANAs are present, nearly always at the time of diagnosis, in essentially 100 percent of patients, although at least one report exists of a child with ANA-negative SLE.[124] ANA tests usually remain consistently positive for years. The patterns of ANA include homogeneous, speckled, and peripheral fluorescence and reactions with specific nuclear antigens such as single-stranded DNA, native DNA, and nucleohistones are similar to those of adults.[40] Antibody to native double-stranded DNA is probably the autoantibody most specific for SLE; Lehman et al. found that high titers of these antibodies correlated with active disease, arthritis, and rash, although not with indicators of active renal disease.[125] As in adults, self-reactive antibodies may be detected against a variety of tissue antigens as well. Anti-red cell antibodies, lymphocytotoxic antibodies, and antineuronal antibodies are only a few examples.

Rheumatoid factors may be present in 5–10 percent of children with SLE, occasionally in high titers. Immunoglobulin levels are usually diffusely elevated. Complement levels, which include CH_{50}, C3, and C4, are usually decreased during active disease and are felt to be good reflectors of disease activity. Singsen et al.[35] found that a wide variety of manifestations of SLE can decrease complement values, and C3 and C4 changes can reflect changes in cutaneous and in CNS disease as well as in renal activity.

Leukopenia is present in about 50 percent of children at the time of diagnosis.[4,10,40] and the frequency of anemia may be even higher. Nonspecific indicators of inflammation, such as the erythrocyte sedimentation rate, are elevated in over 80 percent of children, while a false-positive test for syphilis has been reported in 13–33 percent of children with lupus.[4,6] A positive, direct Coombs test and the presence of circulating anticoagulants are also common in these children.

Overall, DNA binding values and serum complement levels are the most useful parameters of disease activity to follow, but no laboratory test is completely reliable, and each patient must be evaluated individually.

THERAPY

The goals of therapy in childhood SLE should include control of the underlying disease process, attention to specific organ system involvement in the individual child, minimizing the sometimes life-threatening side effects of the treatment itself, and, perhaps most important, providing as normal a life-style as possible for the patient. Thorough evaluation of organ system involvement should be performed before deciding on a particular course of therapy. For that small (5–10 percent) subset of children with mild disease and no renal involvement, aspirin may be used to reduce fever, malaise, and other systemic symptoms. Some authors feel however, that children with SLE may be more susceptible to aspirin-induced hepatotoxicity,[40] although there are no reports of permanent, significant liver dysfunction in this situation. Liver enzymes should be monitored, though, and other nonsteroidal anti-inflammatory drugs (NSAID) may be used if significant abnormalities appear. There are no suggestions at this point that certain NSAIDs may be more efficacious in this setting than any others.

For the majority of other children with more significant disease, corticosteroids are the cornerstone of therapy. Initial high doses (40–60 mg/per/ m^2/day) in divided doses will usually bring the disease under control. After a few weeks with good response the dose should gradually be switched to a single daily dose or an alternate day schedule and then tapered very slowly to the minimum dose that controls symptoms and signs of the disease. Too rapid tapering often leads to recurrence of symptoms and an overall higher steroid requirement. The side effects of continuing high-dose daily steroids can be dangerous and so troublesome as to lead to noncompliance, especially in adolescents; fortunately, prolonged high doses are rarely needed to control the disease process. Often, antimalarials or nonsteroidal anti-inflammatory drugs can be added to reduce the steroid requirement. Hydroxychloroquine is the recommended antimalarial agent, but the possibility of retinal damage requires an ophthalmologic exam before and 3 or 4 times yearly during its administration.

If adequate response cannot be obtained with reasonable steroid dosages, a cytotoxic agent may be considered. Azathioprine, chlorambucil, cyclophosphamide, and nitrogen mustard have all been used in childhood SLE. Studies on their effectiveness and side effects in children are inconclusive, and none is clearly superior to the others.[40] Short-term toxicity centers on severe leukopenia with the attendant danger of sepsis. Long-term side effects include the potential for sterility with chlorambucil and cyclophosphamide and the unproven but presumed higher risk of malignancy with all four. Cyclophosphamide can also lead to hemorrhagic cystitis, which can sometimes recur even after the drug has been discontinued. On the other hand, these agents do not interfere with normal growth and hence may be quite useful when used in combination with corticosteroids.

Adjunctive therapy aimed at specific disease manifestations has probably helped decrease the morbidity and mortality of childhood lupus, too. Antihypertensives should be used where appropriate. Management of cardiac embarrassment, pulmonary dysfunction, fluid and electrolyte balance, and coagulopathies can all be lifesaving. Again, it is always important to think of infection as a cause of fever in childhood lupus. Only thorough evaluation and institution of appropriate therapy will minimize morbidity and mortality from infectious disease in this setting. Hemodialysis and renal transplantation may provide hope for otherwise terminally ill patients.

Less well-established modalities include pulse methylprednisolone therapy, which has been reported to give good results with few side effects in some cases of diffuse proliferative lupus nephritis.[126] Long-term effects of pulse therapy are not yet known.

Plasmapheresis has gained recent attention as an experimental therapy for SLE, but its use in childhood lupus has not been systematically studied.

Finally, the need for attention to the psychological needs of the child cannot be overemphasized. Physical activity need not be restricted in most cases, and school attendance, involvement in extracurricular activities, and career planning should all be encouraged. The child should be involved in all aspects of his or her care as early as possible, and should be encouraged to take responsibility for home care as soon as he or she is old enough. Counseling, by a member of the team or a psychologist or psychiatrist, should be readily available.

DISEASE COURSE AND OUTCOME

As in adult disease, the pattern of childhood lupus is one of recurrent flares and "remissions." Even with appropriate corticosteroid therapy, this course of exacerbations punctuating periods of low-disease activity appears essentially unchanged. In Hanson's study of over 100 children with lupus,[40] he found approximately 5 percent to have mild disease, with only infrequent and noncritical exacerbations. Other children displayed severe disease with significant renal, as well as other organ system, involvement, but after approximately 1 year of aggressive treatment most signs of their disease resolved and they enjoyed often prolonged periods of remission. Much more common, however, was the pattern of low-grade disease activity with frequent serious flares that involved multiple organ systems, any one of which may lead to significant morbidity or even mortality. Unfortunately, there is at this time no way to predict which patients will fall into these subgroups.

The range of complications to which these children are susceptible has been discussed by the organ system above. The recognition and prompt treatment of many of these complications may be responsible for much of the improved morbidity and mortality statistics achieved in recent years. Specifically, the suspicion of infectious disease must always be borne in mind, in untreated patients as well as in those on immunosuppressives. More effective control of hypertension as well as sophisticated intensive care measures and dialysis for those in renal failure have all contributed to better outcomes. The degree to which corticosteroid treatment itself has helped is uncertain, but most would agree that it is a major reason for decreased morbidity and mortality.

Causes of mortality are summarized in Table 2-4. Renal failure and infection together account for over 50 percent of all deaths, while the others are scattered among many causes.

Actual statistics for improved mortality are only estimates. Since Meislin and Rothfield[4] reported in 1968 that childhood lupus had a worse prognosis than adult disease, many other authors have disagreed. But all concur that survival rates are much improved over the past few decades. Hanson reports an approximate 75–85 percent mortality in the first 5 years of disease in 1960, with only a 15–25 percent mortality in 10 years of disease in the 1970s.[40] Other authors corroborate these figures. Norris et al. report a 73 percent mortality rate in children followed before 1960 and a 28 percent mortality in those diagnosed after that year.[9] Caeiro et al. estimate an 82.6 percent 5-year survival rate and 76.7 percent 10-year survival rate for their study of 42 childhood lupus patients.[11] Similarly, Fish et al.[7] report a 10-year survival rate of 86 percent for a group of 49 children, while Walravens and Chase describe a 63 percent survival rate among 50 children diagnosed after 1965.[127] Jacobs[128] divides his childhood patients into groups diagnosed from 1930–1946, 1949–1960, 1961–1967, and 1967–1977; the survival rates for the first 3 years of disease are striking: 0, 43, 63, and 89 percent, respectively.

Division of children into clinical subgroups may provide a better predictor of disease outcome in an individual case. For example, Abeles et al.[129] found a 100 percent 5-year survival among children with membranous or focal lupus nephritis, compared to an 85 percent rate among those with diffuse proliferative nephritis. Similarly, Caeiro et al.'s study found a 5- and 10-year survival rate of 59.5 and 47.5 percent, respectively, in children with lupus nephritis of all types, with no deaths in the nonnephritic group.[11] Interestingly, the same study also estimates a 5-year survival rate for females of 83 percent and for males of 47.5 percent. They caution, however, that this difference was not statistically significant because of the small number of male patients studied.

Table 2-4
Causes of Mortality in Childhood SLE

Reference	Total patients	Total deaths	Renal failure	Infection	Cardiac failure	CNS	Vasculitis	Pulmonary hemorrhage	Pancreatitis	Acute lupus	Transfusion reaction	GI	Hepatic failure	Misc.
			(% of Deaths)											
Meislin and Rothfield[4]	42	18	33	39		11				11			.6	
Garin et al.[62]	49	6	33	33		33								
Kornreich[5]	90	24	46	25			8	12	8					
Walravens and Chase[127]	50	13	33	17	42						.8			.8
Fish et al.[7]	49	7		85					14					
Wallace et al.[10]	45	9	11	44	11	22				22				
Abeles et al.[129]	67	10	30	10			10					10		40
Caeiro et al.[11]	42	6	33	50	17									
Total	434	93	27.4	38.2	9	8.2	2	2	3	4	.1	1	.1	5

In summary, overall survival in childhood lupus has improved greatly in recent years, while renal failure and infection remain important causes of death in younger lupus patients. Statistics for specific clinical subgroups of patients may lead to better predictions of outcome for these children.

NEONATAL LUPUS PHENOMENA

By far the most common problems in pregnancies of women with SLE are an increased risk of miscarriage and low birth weights in live-born infants. Much interest has recently been focused on specific lupus phenomena in some of these infants, however. Most descriptions of "neonatal lupus" can be attributed to passive transfer of maternal autoantibodies, as discussed below. The existence of a separate, distinct clinical entity of neonatal lupus is still uncertain.

Several cases of lupus that occurs in newborns have been reported. One infant, whose mother was thought to be normal, had discoid skin lesions present on her face at birth, which later spread to involve most of her body.[130] She had low-titer ANA and positive LE cells found on a bone marrow specimen obtained at 3 months of age, although no peripheral LE cells were noted. On these bases she was diagnosed as having congenital SLE.

A second patient, also of an asymptomatic mother, was described as having congenital SLE.[131] She had petechiae at birth, with thrombocytopenia, positive Coomb's test, and a positive LE-cell preparation. She continued to have difficulties with hemolytic anemia and died at 4 years of age, presumably from congestive heart failure secondary to her anemia, although no postmortem examination was performed.

Hull et al.[132] reported the findings of an infant who died within minutes of birth, whose mother had had long-standing SLE during pregnancy. The baby had edema, a blotchy purpuric rash, hepatosplenomegaly, and complete heart block. Postmortem findings included a large pericardial effusion, extensive endocardial fibroelastosis, with diffuse fibrosis of heart muscle, liver, spleen, kidneys, and adrenals. No ANA could be detected in a cord blood sample.

A final case involves an infant who also died shortly after birth; his mother had some evidence of SLE (rash, arthritis, leukopenia), but no LE cells could be detected.[133] This infant also had complete heart block, and the most striking findings at autopsy were in the heart: extensive subendocardial fibroelastosis and hematoxylin bodies in the areas of the rings of the AV valves, AV groove, and the right auricular appendage.

These descriptions of congenital systemic lupus erythematosus are intriguing; however, most were not studied completely, and none fulfills current diagnostic criteria for SLE; therefore, existence of this entity awaits further confirmation.

Much more widely recognized is the phenomenon of abnormalities, frequently transient, in infants born to mothers with SLE or other rheumatic diseases. In contrast to the cases mentioned above, these newborns are usually clinically well without life-threatening complications. The findings fall into three main categories: cutaneous, hematologic, and cardiac abnormalities.

The rash of discoid lupus has been the most commonly described cutaneous change in these infants.[134–137] It may occur primarily around the malar eminences and eyes or may extend to include the scalp, trunk, and extremities. In most cases, the eruption shows well-circumscribed, erythematous, scaling lesions but can also become confluent. Telangiectasia are prominent findings. Less frequently, petechiae are present, either localized or generalized. In most cases, the rash is present at birth, but onset can be delayed by as much as 5 weeks.[138]

Histologic changes of these eruptions are in most cases consistent with classic discoid lupus. In general, the epidermis shows atrophic changes with some hyperkeratosis and a varying degree of liquefaction degeneration. The dermis often displays interstitial edema and focal lymphocytic infiltration. Some specimens show thickening of the basement membrane zone; direct immunofluorescence demonstrated IgG and IgM to be present at the dermoepidermal junction in 1 case,[134] whereas in 2 other cases, C3 was demonstrated by the same methods.[139]

In the majority of cases, the rash resolved spontaneously within the first 6 months of life. Epstein and Litt[135] reported a child with rash as the only symptom, whose lesions persisted for 18 months, however, and Brustein et al. have reported 2 children whose discoid lesions continued to ages 11 and 28 months, respectively.[139] No residue remained once the rash resolved, except for mild atrophy and hypopigmentation in a few cases. The differential diagnosis for neonatal discoid lupus, as discussed by Vonderheid et al.,[134] includes Bloom's syndrome, a triad of congenital telangiectatic erythema of the face, photosensitivity, and growth retardation.

A more serious complication for infants of mothers with SLE-like syndromes includes cardiac involvement. Rare cases of subendocardial fibroelastosis have already been mentioned. More common are examples of complete AV heart block.[132–134,140–143] In some cases this is discovered antenatally; it occasionally progresses to heart failure and hydrops fetalis.[140] In one review of 31 cases of congenital heart block associated with maternal connective tissue disease, Hardy et al.[144] reported a mortality rate of 29 percent; approximately 50 percent of these children died in the immediate perinatal period and 50 percent died later in childhood, with 2 of them developing cardiomyopathies just prior to death. Six of these 31 infants had associated cardiac anomalies; this included patent ductus arteriosus and transposition of the great vessels. In a few cases, treatment with digoxin or insertion of a pacemaker became necessary. Most often, however, the heart block requires no therapy and the child is clinically well.

Many have speculated that transplacental passage of maternal antibodies may be responsible for the condition. McCue et al.[142] suggest that the collagen framework around the SA and the AV nodes may be particularly susceptible to abnormal maternal antibodies. This intriguing possibility awaits further study.

The overall incidence of congenital complete heart block is quite small, but when the mothers of all children with this condition are evaluated, 30–50 percent of them have evidence of connective tissue disease, most commonly SLE.[142,143,145] It is interesting to note that frequently the birth of an affected child precedes the diagnosis in the mother; this prompts one to study and closely monitor these mothers for development of disease. Many examples exist of more than one affected sibling born to a mother with SLE.[142,143,146]

Finally, Doshi et al. have recently described a single case of congenital pericarditis due to maternal SLE.[147] The infant was stillborn, and postmortem examination revealed extensive fibrinous pericarditis with thick granulation tissue and marked capillary proliferation. ANA studies performed on heart blood were positive in high titer.

Hematologic abnormalities may also occur in infants of mothers with SLE. Hemolytic anemia, leukopenia, and thrombocytopenia have all been described and are usually transient and asymptomatic,[131,134,148,149] although at least 1 patient had persistent hemolytic anemia lasting several years until her death.[131] Some infants of SLE mothers show other serologic abnormalities such as ANAs, but one recent report found positive ANAs or LE cells in only 9 of 23 infants.[138] A recent report has demonstrated the presence of anti-Ro (SSA) and anti-La (SSB) antibodies in an ANA-negative neonate with discoid lupus; his asymptomatic mother had the same serologic pattern.[150] These transiently positive lupus markers are presumed to be due to passive placental transfer of these factors from the maternal circulation. Similarly, most of the hematologic abnormalities are postulated to be due to maternal antibodies against red blood cells, platelets, etc. Nathan and Snapper demonstrated placental transfer of factors that lead to thrombocytopenia and the LE phenomenon as early as 1958.[149] Again, this explanation, although quite attractive, has yet to be proven.

What is then the overall outcome of infants born to mothers with SLE? The occurrence of fetal wastage is quite high in lupus, approximately 30 percent by some estimates. Of live-born infants, however, 50–75 percent are apparently completely normal. Another 10 percent or so have transient hematologic or serologic abnormalities, which resolve spontaneously in most cases. Of those with discoid lupus lesions and no other involvement, again the course is usually spontaneous resolution with minimal residua. Cardiac involvement obviously carries the highest risk; as mentioned, up to 30 percent may die by early childhood. Finally, 2 cases of infants of mothers with SLE were described who were born with transient discoid lesions but who developed classical systemic lupus at a much later age (13 and 19 years, respectively).[151,152]

SUMMARY

SLE in children is similar to that in adults. One significant difference is the paucity of mild cases of SLE in children; 95 percent have serious, often life-threatening complications at some point during their course, which require close follow-up. Diagnosis of SLE in very young patients should raise one's suspicions of associated factors, such as complement deficiencies or anticonvulsant use. Similarly, evidence of lupus in newborns should prompt one to search for rheumatic disease in the mother.

Corticosteroid administration is still the cornerstone of therapy; aggressive therapy of the basic disease as well as prompt treatment of multisystem complications and careful attention to the side effects of treatment, particularly infections and interference with growth, has led to improved outcome in recent years; this allows an optimistic outlook for long-term survival and a reasonably normal lifestyle in most of these children.

REFERENCES

1. Cook, CD, Wedgwood RJ, Craig JM, et al.: Systemic lupus erythematosus: Description of 37 cases in children and discussion of endocrine therapy in 32 of the cases. Pediatrics 26:570–585, 1960
2. Jacobs JC: Systemic lupus erythematosus in childhood: Report of 35 cases, with discussion of 7 apparently induced by convulsant medication and of prognosis and treatment. Pediatrics 32:257–264, 1963
3. Robinson MJ, Williams AL: Systemic lupus erythematosus in childhood. Aust Paediatr J 3:36–47, 1967
4. Meislin AG, Rothfield N: Systemic lupus erythematosus in childhood: Analysis of 42 cases with comparative data on 200 adult cases followed concurrently. Pediatrics 42:37–49, 1968
5. Kornreich H: Systemic lupus erythematosus in childhood. Clin Rheum Dis 2:429–443, 1976
6. Coleman WP III, Coleman WP, Derbes VJ, et al.: Collagen disease in children: A review of 71 cases. JAMA 237:1095–1100, 1977
7. Fish AJ, Blau EB, Westberg NG, et al.: Systemic lupus erythematosus within the first two decades of life. Am J Med 62:99–117, 1977
8. King KK, Kornreich HK, Bernstein BH, et al.: The clinical spectrum of systemic lupus erythematosus in childhood. Arthritis Rheum 20:287–294, 1977
9. Norris DG, Colon AR, Stickler GB: Systemic lupus erythematosus in children: The complex problems of diagnosis and treatment encountered in 101 such patients at the Mayo Clinic. Clin Ped (Phila) 16:774–778, 1977
10. Wallace C, Schaller JG, Emery H, et al.: Prospective study of childhood systemic lupus erythematosus (SLE). Arthritis Rheum 21:599–600, 1978
11. Caeiro F, Michielson FMC, Bernstein R, et al.: Systemic lupus erythematosus in childhood. Ann Rheum Dis 40:325–331, 1981
12. Schaller JG: Lupus in childhood. Clin Rheum Dis 8:219–228, 1982
13. Tan EM, Cohen AS, Fries JF, et al.: The 1982 revised criteria for the classification of systemic lupus erythematosus. Arthritis Rheum 25:1271–1277, 1982
14. Block SR, Winfield JB, Lockshin MD, et al.: Studies of twins with systemic lupus erythematosus: A review of the literature and presentation of 12 additional sets. Am J Med 59:533–552, 1975

15. Arnett FC, Shulman LE: Studies in familial systemic lupus erythematosus. Medicine 55:313–322, 1976
16. Koroleva NI, Kaladze NN, Kirichenko A: Collagen disease in twins (Russian). Voprosy Reumatiza 13:53–55, 1973
17. Lowenstein MB, Rothfield NF: Family study of systemic lupus erythematosus: Analysis of the clinical history, skin immunofluorescence, and serologic parameters. Arthritis Rheum 20:1293–1303, 1977
18. DeHoratius RJ, Messner RD: Lymphocytotoxic antibodies in family members of patients with systemic lupus erythematosus. J Clin Invest 55:1254–1258, 1975.
19. Malave I, Papa R, Layrisse A: Lymphocytotoxic Antibodies in SLE Patients and their relatives. Arthritis Rheum 19:700–704, 1976
20. Lehman TJA, Hanson V, Singsen BH, et al.: Serum complement abnormalities in ANA positive relatives of children with SLE. Arthritis Rheum 22:954–958, 1979
21. Buckman KJ, Moore SK, Ebbin AJ, et al.: Familial systemic lupus erythematosus. Arch Intern Med 138:1674–1676, 1978
22. Schur PH, Meyer I, Garovoy M, et al.: Associations between systemic lupus erythematosus and the major histocompatibility complex: Clinical and immunological considerations. Clin Immunol Immunopathol 24:263–273, 1982
23. Scherak O, Smolen JS, Mayr WR: HLA-DRw 3 and systemic lupus erythematosus. Arthritis Rheum 23:954–957, 1980
24. Bell DA, Maddison PJ: Serologic subsets in systemic lupus erythematosus: An examination of autoantibodies in relationship to clinical features of disease and HLA antigens. Arthritis Rheum 23:1268–1273, 1980
25. Cleland LG, Bell DA, Willans M, et al.: Familial lupus: Family studies of HLA and serologic findings. Arthritis Rheum 21:183–191, 1978
26. Black CM, Welsh KI, Fielder A, et al.: HLA antigens and Bf allotypes in SLE: Evidence for the association being with specific haplotypes. Tissue Antigens 19:115–120, 1982
27. Day NK, Geiger H, McLain R, et al.: C2 deficiency: Development of lupus erythematosus. J Clin Invest 52:1601–1607, 1973
28. Schaller JG, Gilliland BG, Ochs HD, et al.: Severe systemic lupus erythematosus with nephritis in a boy with deficiency of the fourth component of complement. Arthritis Rheum 20:1519–1525, 1977
29. Moncada B, Day NK, Good RA, et al.: Lupus erythematosus-like syndrome with a familial defect of complement. N Engl Med 286:689–693, 1972
30. Agnello V, deBracco ME, Kunkel HG: Hereditary C2 deficiency with some manifestations of systemic lupus erythematosus. J Immunol 108:837–840, 1972
31. Ballow M, McLean RH, Einerson M, et al.: Hereditary C4 deficiency-genetic studies and linkage to HLA. Transplant Proc 11:1710–1712, 1979
32. Gewurz A, Lint TF, Roberts JL, et al.: Homozygous C2 deficiency with fulminant lupus erythematosus. Arthritis Rheum 21:28–36, 1978
33. Glass D, Raum D, Gibson D, et al.: Inherited deficiency of the second component of complement. J. Clin Invest 58:853–861, 1976.
34. Petty RE, Palmer NR, Cassidy JT, et al.: The association of autoimmune diseases and anti-IgA antibodies in patients with selective IgA deficiency. Clin Exp Immunol 37:83–88, 1979
35. Singsen BH, Fishman L, Hanson V: Antinuclear antibodies and lupus-like syndromes in children receiving anticonvulsants. Pediatrics 57:529–534, 1976
36. Beernick DH, Miller JJ III: Anticonvulsant induced antinuclear antibodies and lupus-like disease in children. J Pediatr 82:113–117, 1973
37. Fessel WJ: Systemic lupus erythematosus in the community. Arch Intern Med 134:1027–1035, 1974
38. Grossman J, Schwartz RH, Callerame ML, et al.: Systemic lupus erythematosis in a 1-year-old child. Am J Dis Child 129:123–125, 1975
39. Rothfield N: Clinical features of SLE, in Kelley WN, Harris ED, Ruddy S, Sledge CB (eds): Textbook of Rheu-

matology. Philadelphia, W. B. Saunders, 1981
40. Hanson V: Systemic lupus erythematosus, dermatomyositis, scleroderma, and vasculitides in childhood, in Kelley WN, Harris ED, Ruddy S, Sledge CB (eds): Textbook of Rheumatology. Philadelphia, W. B. Saunders, 1981
41. Tuffanelli DL, Dubois EL: Cutaneous manifestations of systemic lupus erythematosus. Arch Dermatol 90:377–386, 1964
42. Furey NL, Esterly NB: Lupus erythematosus, in Solomon CM, Esterly NB, Loeffel ED (eds): Adolescent Dermatology, Major Problems in Clinical Pediatrics, Vol. 19. Philadelphia, W. B. Saunders, 1978
43. Gilliam JN, Sontheimer RD: Distinctive cutaneous subsets in the spectrum of lupus erythematosus (editorial). J Am Acad Dermatol 4:471–475, 1981
44. Sotor NA: The skin in individuals with lupus erythematosus. J Rheumatol 7:392–395, 1980
45. Koransky JS, Esterly NB: Lupus panniculitis (profundus). J Pediatr 98:241–244, 1981
46. Budman DR, Steinberg AD: Hematologic aspects of systemic lupus erythematosus: Current concepts. Ann Intern Med 86:220–229, 1977
47. Scott JP, Schiff DW, Githens JH: The autoerythrocyte sensitization syndrome as the primary manifestation of systemic lupus erythematosus. J Pediatr 99:598–600, 1981
48. Hashimoto Y, Ziff M, Hurd ER: Increased endothelial cell adherence, aggregation, and superoxide generation by neutrophils incubated in systemic lupus erythematosus and Felty's syndrome sera. Arthritis Rheum 25:1409–1417, 1982
49. Rivero SJ, Diaz-Jouanen E, Alarcon-Segovia D: Lymphopenia in systemic lupus erythematosus: Clinical, diagnostic, and prognostic significance. Arthritis Rheum 21:295–305, 1978
50. Mittal KK, Rossen RD, Sharp JT, et al.: Lymphocyte cytotoxic antibodies in systemic lupus erythematosus. Nature 225:1255–1256, 1970
51. Messner RP, Kennedy MS, Jelinek JG: Antilymphocyte antibodies in systemic lupus erythematosus. Arthritis Rheum 18:201–206, 1975
52. Winfield JB, Winchester RJ, Kunkel HG: Association of cold-reactive antilymphocyte antibodies with lymphopenia in systemic lupus erythematosus. Arthritis Rheum 18:587–594, 1975
53. Margolius A Jr, Jackson DP, Ratnoff OD: Circulating Anticoagulants. A study of 40 cases and a review of the literature. Medicine (Baltimore) 40:145–202, 1961
54. Schleider MA, Nachman RL, Jaffe EA, et al.: A clinical study of the lupus anticoagulant. Blood 48:499–506, 1976
55. Alger M, Alarcon-Segovia D, Rivero SJ: Hemolytic anemia and thrombocytopenic purpura: Two related subsets of systemic lupus erythematosus. J Rheumatol 4:351–357, 1977
56. Cassidy JT, Sullivan DB, Petty RE, et al.: Lupus nephritis and encephalopathy: Prognosis in 58 children. Arthritis Rheum 20:315–322, 1977
57. Morris MC, Cameron JS, Chantler C, et al.: Systemic lupus erythematosus with nephritis. Arch Dis Child 56:779–783, 1981
58. Miceli LA, Moore ES: Systemic lupus erythematosus: A renal review with a pediatric perspective. JAOA 78:799–808, 1979
59. Garin EH, Shulman ST, Donnelly WH, et al.: Systemic lupus erythematosus glomerulonephritis in children. Pediatrician 10:351–367, 1981
60. Wallace C, Striker G, Schaller JG, et al.: Renal histology and subsequent course in childhood systemic lupus erythematosus (SLE). Arthritis Rheum 20:669, 1979
61. Libit SA, Burke B, Michael AF, et al.: Extramembranous glomerulonephritis in childhood: Relationship to systemic lupus erythematosus. J Pediatr 88:394–402, 1976
62. Garin EH, Donnelly WH, Fennell RS, et al.: Nephritis in systemic lupus erythematosus in children. J Pediatr 89:366–371, 1976
63. Mahajan SK, Ordonez NG, Spargo BH, et al.: Changing histopathology patterns

in lupus nephropathy. Clin Nephrol 10:1–8, 1978
64. Cameron JS, Turner DR, Ogg CS, et al.: Systemic lupus with nephritis: A long-term study. QJ Med 48:1–24, 1979
65. Comerford FR, Cohen AF: Nephropathy of systemic lupus erythematosus: An assessment by clinical, light and electron microscopic criteria. Medicine 46:425–473, 1967
66. Mahajan SK, Ordonez NG, Feitelson PJ, et al.: Lupus nephropathy without clinical renal involvement. Medicine 56:493–501, 1977
67. Woolf A, Croker B, Osofsky SG, et al.: Nephritis in children and young adults with systemic lupus erythematosus and normal urinary sediment. Pediatrics 64:678–685, 1979
68. Weis LS, Pachman LM, Potter EV, et al.: Occult lupus nephropathy: A correlated light, electron, and immunofluorescent microscopic study. Histopathology 1:401–419, 1977
69. Ragsdale CG, Petty RE, Cassidy JT, et al.: The clinical progression of apparent juvenile rheumatoid arthritis to systemic lupus erythematosus. J Rheumatol 7:50–55, 1980
70. Tsokos GC, Moutsopoulos HM, Steinberg AD: Muscle involvement in systemic lupus erythematosus. JAMA 246:766–768, 1981
71. Foote RA, Kimbrough SM, Stevens JC: Lupus myositis. Muscle Nerve 5:65–68, 1982
72. Dubois EL, Cozen L: Avascular (aseptic) bone necrosis associated with systemic lupus erythematosus. JAMA 174:966–971, 1960
73. Griffiths ID, Maini RN, Scott JJ: Clinical and radiological features of osteonecrosis in systemic lupus erythematosus. Ann Rheum Dis 38:413–422, 1979
74. Abeles M, Urman JD, Rothfield NF: Aseptic necrosis of bone in systemic lupus erythematosus: Relationship to corticosteroid therapy. Arch Intern Med 138:750–754, 1978
75. Hurley RM, Steinberg RH, Patriquin H, et al.: Avascular necrosis of the femoral head in childhood systemic lupus erythematosus. CMA Journal 111:781–784, 1974
76. Bergstein JM, Wiens C, Fish AJ, et al.: Avascular necrosis of bone in systemic lupus erythematosus. J Pediatr 85:31–35, 1974
77. Urman JD, Abeles M, Houghton AN, et al.: Aseptic necrosis presenting as wrist pain in SLE. Arthritis Rheum 20:825–828, 1977
78. Vroninks P, Remans J, Kahn MF, et al.: Aseptic bony necrosis in systemic lupus erythematosus: Report of 7 new cases (French). Sem Hop Paris 48:3001–3009, 1972
79. Velayos EE, Leidholt JD, Smyth CJ, et al.: Arthropathy associated with steroid therapy. Ann Intern Med 64:759–771, 1966
80. Smith FE, Sweet DE, Brunner CM, et al.: Avascular necrosis in SLE: An apparent predilection for young patients. Ann Rheum Dis 35:227–232, 1976
81. Collins RL, Turner RA, Nomeir AM, et al.: Cardiopulmonary manifestations of systemic lupus erythematosus. J Rheumatol 5:299–306, 1978
82. Ito M, Kagiyama Y, Omura I, et al.: Cardiovascular manifestations in systemic lupus erythematosus. Jpn Circ J 43:985–994, 1979
83. Cohen AS, Canoso JJ: Pericarditis in the Rheumatologic Diseases. Cardiovasc Clin 7:237–255, 1976
84. Jacobson EJ, Reza MJ: Constrictive pericarditis in systemic lupus erythematosus: Demonstration of immunoglobulins in the pericardium. Arthritis Rheum 21:972–974, 1978.
85. Paget SA, Bulkley BH, Grauer LE, et al.: Mitral valve disease of systemic lupus erythematosus: A cause of severe congestive heart failure reversed by valve replacement. Am J Med 59:134–139, 1975
86. Ishikawa S, Segar WE, Gilbert EF, et al.: Myocardial infarct in a child with systemic lupus erythematosus. Am J Dis Child 132:696–699, 1978
87. Meller J, Conde CA, Deppisch LM, et al.: Myocardial infarction due to coronary atherosclerosis in three young adults with systemic lupus erythematosus. Am J Cardiol 35:309–314, 1975
88. Homcy CJ, Liberthson RR, Fallon JT, et al.: Ischemic heart disease in systemic lupus erythematosus in the young

patient: Report of six cases. Am J Cardiol 49:478–484, 1982

89. Haider VS, Roberts WC: Coronary arterial disease in systemic lupus erythematosus: Quantification of degrees of narrowing in 22 necropsy patients (21 women) aged 16 to 37 years. Am J Med 70:775–781, 1981
90. del Rio A, Vazquez JJ, Sobrino JA, et al.: Myocardial involvement in systemic lupus erythematosus: A noninvasive study of left ventricular function. Chest 74:414–417, 1978
91. Bharati S, de la Fuente DJ, Kallen RJ, et al.: Conduction system in systemic lupus erythematosus with atrioventricular block. Am J Cardiol 35:299–304, 1975
92. Wray R, Iveson M: Complete heart block and systemic lupus erythematosus. Br Heart J 37:982–983, 1975
93. Bidani AK, Roberts JL, Schwartz MM, et al.: Immunopathology of cardiac lesions in fatal systemic lupus erythematosus. Am J Med 69:849–858, 1980
94. Silberstein SL, Barland P, Grayzel AI, et al.: Pulmonary dysfunction in systemic lupus erythematosus: Prevalence classification and correlation with other organ involvement. J Rheumatol 7:187–195, 1980
95. Arnalich F, Ruiz de Andres S, Gil A, et al.: Pulmonary function in systemic lupus erythematosus patients without respiratory symptoms. Bull Europ Physiopath Resp 15:649–657, 1979
96. Fayemi AO: The lung in systemic lupus erythematosus: A clinico-pathologic study of 20 cases. Mount Sinai J Med 42:110–118, 1975
97. Grennan DM, Howie AD, Moran F, et al.: Pulmonary involvement in systemic lupus erythematosus. Ann Rheum Dis 37:536–539, 1978
98. Haupt HM, Moore GW, Hutchins GM: The lung in systemic lupus erythematosus: Analysis of the pathologic changes in 120 patients. Am J Med 71:791–798, 1981
99. Ilowite N, Schaller JG: Unilateral pleural effusions in childhood lupus. 1983 (submitted for publication)
100. Reda MG, Baigelman W: Pleural effusion in systemic lupus erythematosus. Acta Cytol (Baltimore) 24:553–557, 1980
101. Halla JT, Schrohenloher RE, Volanakis JE: Immune complexes and other laboratory features of pleural effusions: A comparison of rheumatoid arthritis, systemic lupus erythematosus, and other diseases. Ann Intern Med 92:748–752, 1980
102. Marino CT, Pertschuk LP: Pulmonary hemorrhage in systemic lupus erythematosus. Arch Intern Med 141:201–203, 1981
103. Eagan JW, Memoli VA, Roberts JL, et al.: Pulmonary hemorrhage in systemic lupus erythematosus. Medicine 57:545–560, 1978
104. Rajani KB, Ashbacher LV, Kinney TR: Pulmonary hemorrhage and systemic lupus erythematosus. J Pediatr 93:810–812, 1978
105. Yancey CL, Doughty RA, Athreya BH: Central nervous system involvement in childhood systemic lupus erythematosus. Arthritis Rheum 24:1389–1395, 1981
106. Bennahum DA, Messner RP: Recent observations on central nervous system systemic lupus erythematosus. Semin Arthritis Rheum 4:253–266, 1975
107. Zeller W: Case records of the Massachusetts General Hospital: N Engl J Med 225:549–552, 1941
108. Kukla LF, Reddy C, Silkalns G, et al.: Systemic lupus erythematosus presenting as chorea. Arch Dis Child 53:345–347, 1978
109. Herd JK, Medhi M, Uzendoski DM, et al.: Chorea associated with systemic lupus erythematosus: Report of two cases and review of the literature. Pediatrics 61:308–315, 1978
110. Sergent JS, Lockshin MD, Klempner MS, et al.: Central nervous system disease in systemic lupus erythematosus: Therapy and prognosis. Am J Med 58:644–654, 1975
111. Feinglass EJ, Arnett FC, Dorsch CA, et al.: Neuropsychiatric manifestations of systemic lupus erythematosus: Diagnosis, clinical spectrum, and relationship to other features of the disease. Medicine 55:323–339, 1976

112. Dubois EL, Wierzchowiecki M, Cox BB, et al.: Duration and death in systemic lupus erythematosus: Analysis of 249 cases. JAMA 227:1399–1402, 1974
113. Hoffman BI, Katz WA: The gastrointestinal manifestations of systemic lupus erythematosus: A review of the literature. Semin Arthritis Rheum 9:237–247, 1980
114. Reynolds JC, Inman RD, Kimberly RP, et al.: Acute pancreatitis in systemic lupus erythematosus: Report of twenty cases and a review of the literature. Medicine 61:25–32, 1982
115. Runyon BA, LaBrecque DR, Anuras S: The spectrum of liver disease in systemic lupus erythematosus: Report of 33 histologically-proved cases and review of the literature. Am J Med 69:187–194, 1980
116. Ropes MW: Systemic Lupus Erythematosus. Cambridge, Harvard Univ. Press, 1976
117. Hermann G: Intussusception secondary to mesenteric arteritis: Complication of systemic lupus erythematosus in a 5-year-old-child. JAMA 200:74–75, 1967
118. Binstadt DH, L'Heureux PR: Pneumatosis cystoides intestinalis in childhood systemic lupus erythematosus. Minn Med 60:408–409, 1977
119. Matolo NM, Albo D Jr: Gastrointestinal complications of collagen vascular diseases: Surgical implications. Am J Surg 122:678–682, 1971
120. Tsukahara M, Matsuo K, Kojima H: Protein-losing enteropathy in a boy with systemic lupus erythematosus. J Pediatr 97:778–780, 1980
121. Ramirez-Mata M, Reyes PA, Alarcon-Segovia D, et al.: Esophageal motility in systemic lupus erythematosus. Am J Dig Dis 19:132–136, 1974
122. Lessell S: Some ophthalmologic and neurologic aspects of systemic lupus erythematosus. J Rheum 7:398–404, 1980
123. Richards GE, Pachman LM, Green OC: Symptomatic hypothyroidism in children with collagen disease. J Pediatr 87:82–84, 1975
124. Gillespie JP, Lindsley CB, Linshaw MA, et al.: Childhood systemic lupus erythematosus with negative antinuclear antibody test. J Pediatr 98:578–581, 1981
125. Lehman TJA, Hanson V, Singsen BH, et al.: The role of antibodies directed against double-stranded DNA in the manifestations of systemic lupus erythematosus in childhood. J Pediatr 96:657–661, 1980
126. Barron KS, Person DA, Brewer EJ, et al.: Pulse methylprednisolone therapy in diffuse proliferative lupus nephritis. J Pediatr 101:137–141, 1982
127. Walravens PA, Chase HP: The prognosis of childhood systemic lupus erythematosus. Am J Dis Child 130:929–933, 1976
128. Jacobs JC: Childhood-onset systemic lupus erythematosus: Modern management and improved prognosis. NY State J Med 77:2231–2233, 1977
129. Abeles M, Urman JD, Weinstein A, et al.: Systemic lupus erythematosus in the younger patient: Survival studies. J Rheumatol 7:515–523, 1980
130. East WR, Lumpkin LR: Systemic lupus erythamatosus in the newborn. Minn Med 52:477–478, 1969
131. Nice CM Jr: Congenital disseminated lupus erythematosus. Am J Roentgenol 88:585–587, 1962
132. Hull D, Binns BAO, Joyce D: Congenital heart block and widespread fibrosis due to maternal lupus erythematosus. Arch Dis Child 41:688–690, 1966
133. Hogg GR: Congenital, acute lupus erythematosus associated with subendocardial fibroelastosis: Report of a case. Am J Clin Pathol 28:648–654, 1957
134. Vonderheid EC, Koblenzer PJ, Ming PML, et al.: Neonatal lupus erythematosus. Arch Dermatol 112:698–705, 1976
135. Epstein HC, Litt JZ: Discoid lupus erythematosus in a newborn infant. N Engl J Med 265:1106–1107, 1961
136. McCuiston CH, Schoch EP Jr: Possible discoid LE in newborn infant: Report of a case with subsequent development of SLE in mother. Arch Dermatol 70:782–785, 1954
137. Bremers HH, Golitz LE, Weston WL, et al.: Neonatal lupus erythematosus. Cutis 24:287–290, 1979
138. Draznin TH, Esterly NB, Furey NL, et al.: Neonatal lupus erythematosus. J Am Acad Dermatol 1:437–442, 1979

139. Brustein D, Rodriguez JM, Minkin W, et al.: Familial lupus erythematosus. JAMA 238:2294–2295, 1977
140. Altenburger KM, Jedziniak M, Roper WL, et al.: Congenital complete heart block associated with hydrops fetalis. J Pediatr 91:618–620, 1977
141. Chameides L, Truex RC, Vetter V, et al.: Association of maternal systemic lupus erythematosus with congenital complete heart block. N Engl J Med 297:1204–1207, 1977
142. McCue CM, Mantakas ME, Tingelstad JB, et al.: Congenital heart block in newborns of mothers with connective tissue disease. Circulation 56:82–90, 1977
143. Esscher E, Scott JS: Congenital heart block and maternal systemic lupus erythematosus. Br Med J 1:1235–1238, 1979
144. Hardy JD, Solomon S, Banwell GS, et al.: Congenital complete heart block in the newborn associated with maternal systemic lupus erythematosus and other connective tissue disorders. Arch Dis Child 54:7–13, 1979
145. Schaller JG, Wallace C, Stamm S, et al.: The occurrence of congenital heart block in infants of mothers with clinical or serological evidence of rheumatic disease. Arthritis Rheum 20:656, 1979 (abstract)
146. Winkler RB, Nora AH, Nora JJ: Familial congenital complete heart block and maternal systemic lupus erythematosus. Circulation 56:1103–1107, 1977
147. Doshi N, Smith B, Klionsky B: Congenital pericarditis due to maternal lupus erythematosus. J Pediatr 96:699–701, 1980
148. Seip M: Systemic lupus erythematosus in pregnancy with hemolytic anemia, leukopenia and thrombocytopenia in the mother and her newborn infant. Arch Dis Child 35:364–366, 1960
149. Nathan DJ, Snapper I: Simultaneous placental transfer of factors responsible for LE formation and thrombocytopenia. Am J Med 25:647–653, 1958
150. Kephart DC, Hood AF, Provost TT: Neonatal lupus erythematosus: New serologic findings. J Invest Dermatol 77:331–333, 1981
151. Jackson R, Gulliver M: Neonatal lupus erythematosus progressing into systemic lupus erythematosus: A 15 year follow-up. Br J Dermatol 101:81–86, 1979
152. Fox RJ, McCuiston CH, Schoch EP: Systemic lupus erythematosus: Association with previous neonatal lupus erythematosus. Arch Dermatol 115:340, 1979

M. Bashar Kahaleh
E. Carwile LeRoy

3

Scleroderma (Systemic Sclerosis): Treatment and Clinical Manifestations as Related to Pathogenesis

GENERAL CHARACTERISTICS

Definition

Scleroderma (systemic sclerosis) is a multisystem disease of unknown etiology that is characterized by inflammatory, vascular, and fibrotic changes of skin and certain internal organs, *VIZ.*, the gastrointestinal tract, lungs, heart, and kidneys. Individual patients with scleroderma show a wide variety of organ involvement and widely variable rates of disease progression (Table 3-1). Localized forms of scleroderma (morphea, linear scleroderma, coup de sabre, etc.) are characterized by patchy fibrosis limited to the skin and structures immediately adjacent to the skin; almost without exception, these localized forms are not associated with visceral disease and will not be discussed here. The systemic form evolves in unpredictable and multiple stages; the clinical expression of each stage varies in severity from mild and slowly progressive to severe and rapidly evolving. Attempts to define subgroups of patients with scleroderma (e.g., CREST syndrome [an often confusing acronym derived from the clinical features: Calcinosis, Raynaud's phenomenon, Esophageal hypomotility, Sclerodactyly, and Telangectasias] and/or acrosclerosis) for purposes of prognosis have not been entirely satisfactory.[1] Also, the concept that the disorder is uniformly progressive (i.e., progressive systemic sclerosis) does not take into account those patients whose cutaneous involvement remains stable or improves spontaneously.[2]

PROGRESS IN CLINICAL RHEUMATOLOGY VOL. I ISBN 0-8089-1646-7

Table 3-1
Classification of Scleroderma

- Generalized scleroderma (systemic sclerosis)
  - Diffuse scleroderma (acute and chronic)
  - CREST syndrome (calcinosis, Raynaud's phenomenon, esophageal hypomotility, sclerodactyly, telangiectasia)
- Localized scleroderma
  - Morphea
  - Linear scleroderma
- Scleroderma-like syndromes
  - Occupational
    - Vinyl chloride associated
    - Vibration associated ("jackhammer disease")
    - Silicosis associated
  - Fasciitis with eosinophilia
  - Scleredemaasis of Buschke (often postinfectious)
  - Metabolic
    - Porphyria
    - Amyloid
  - Immunologic
    - Graft-versus-host reaction
- Scleroderma-associated syndromes
  - Overlap or mixed connective tissue syndromes
    - Sclerolupus
    - Sclerodermatomyositis
    - Scleromyxedema
    - Primary biliary cirrhosis
    - Sjögren's syndrome
  - Inherited
    - Werner's syndrome
    - Phenylketonuria
    - Brandywine triracial isolate
  - Tumor-associated
    - Carcinoid syndrome
    - Bronchoalveolar carcinoma

Adapted from LeRoy EC: Scleroderma (systemic sclerosis), in Kelley WN, Harris ED Jr. Ruddy S. Sledge CB, (eds): Textbook of Rheumatology. Philadelphia, W. B. Saunders, 1981. With permission.

Early stages of scleroderma consist of vascular instability (Raynaud's phenomenon) followed after months to years by a puffy edematous stage which, in turn, evolves into a fibrotic stage. This cycle recurs at various sites at different rates; a patient may have hidebound skin on the hands and puffy skin on the forearms; this raises fundamental problems of early diagnosis, differential diagnosis, assessment of disease activity and prognosis, evaluation of therapy, and validity of interseries comparisons. It is crucial to consider each stage of scleroderma separately with regard to the particular system suspected of involvement.

Taut skin proximal to the metacarpophalangeal joint has been identified as the major diagnostic criterion for scleroderma.[3] This same cooperative study identified sclerodactyly, digital pitting scars, and bilateral basilar pulmonary interstitial markings on chest roentgenogram as minor criteria. The major criterion alone or two minor criteria document a diagnosis of scleroderma. Scleroderma-like syndromes have been described in individuals exposed to vinyl chloride, the antitumor drug bleomycin, and pentazocine. Patients with chronic graft-versus-host reactions may develop a scleroderma-like syndrome. Animal models for scleroderma have been described; they are imperfect replicas of the human disease.[4,5]

Components of scleroderma seen in other connective tissue diseases include sclerodactyly, Raynaud's phenomenon, telangiectasias, esophageal hypomotility, interstitial lung disease, and inflammatory myositis.[6] These (overlap syndromes) are seen particularly in dermatomyositis (sclerodermatomyositis), systemic lupus erythematosus, and rheumatoid arthritis.

Epidemiology

Scleroderma is more common in women than in men, especially in the child-bearing years, which suggests important sex-and-age-related factors in its occurrence.[7] The disease, rare in children, increases steadily with age. No strong racial predilection is found in males, but the disease seems to be more frequent in black females than in white females. Familial cases are being reported with increasing frequency, but no consistent genetic factors have been identified. The estimated incidence of scleroderma varies from 1/10,000/yr to 1/100,000/yr.[7]

Early Detection

In the majority of cases, the disease starts with Raynaud's phenomenon; this continues for months to years before hidebound skin changes or visceral involvement make the diagnosis of scleroderma obvious. Raynaud's phenomenon defines an episodic constriction of small arteries and arterioles of the fingers, toes, and, occasionally, the face in response to cold or emotional stimuli. The episodes are characterized by triphasic segmental color changes, which consist of pallor, cyanosis, and rubor. One or more of these color changes may be observed in individual patients. Numbness and stiffness usually occur during the phases of pallor and cyanosis. Pain and tingling are often experienced during the phase of rubor. On examination, the fingers may be abnormally cool (particularly if the process has been severe or prolonged). There may be ulceration at the tips of the digits or scars of healed ulceration. At times, this may manifest as flattening or concavity of the distal finger pulp. There may also be loss of hair over the proximal phalanx and tightness of the skin over the distal fingers dorsally (sclerodactyly). The toes and, occasionally, the nose or ears may be similarly involved.

The major clinical challenge in patients with Raynaud's phenomenon is to select those destined to develop scleroderma, systemic lupus erythematosus, or other connective tissue disorders at the earliest possible stage in the patient's illness. The detection of the earliest stages of scleroderma begins with the recognition of Raynaud's phenomenon and puffy hands. Patients may also note fatigue and lack of energy. The "puffy-hand" syndrome can be seen as an early feature not only of scleroderma but also of systemic lupus erythematosus, dermatomyositis, rheumatoid arthritis, and certain subsets of vasculitis. All such patients should be designated as undifferentiated until such time as they evolve into a classic rheumatic syndrome.[8] The presence of antibodies to double-stranded DNA or to Sm antigen favors systemic lupus erythematosus, while erosive arthritis favors rheumatoid arthritis. At present, the most promising prescleroderma features are morphological and flow abnormalities of the cutaneous microvascular bed (scleroderma-pattern capillaries) and the presence of anticentromere antibodies.[9] Morphologic studies of nailfold capillaries with widefield capillary microscopy in scleroderma led to the recognition of scleroderma-specific capillary patterns; these consist of enlarged capillary loops, loss of capillaries, and disruption of the orderly appearance of capillary beds.[10] In a prospective study of Raynaud's phenomenon, capillary changes, as well as serum antinuclear antibodies (ANAs), were found to be associated with future development of connective tissue disease, particularly scleroderma.[11]

Natural History

Although the course of scleroderma is variable, once significant visceral involvement occurs, a fatal outcome from the disease is usual. Using life-table analyses, 5-year survivals range from 36–73 percent. Poor survival is seen in men, in older patients, and in black females. Involvement of the kidney, heart, or lungs are the worst prognostic signs in decreasing order; they act independently of one another. Severe skin involvement is associated with decreased survival because of its association with visceral involvement. The course of the CREST syndrome is slower but otherwise not significantly different from that of diffuse scleroderma.[7]

CLINICAL FEATURES

Skin Involvement

Cutaneous involvement is the hallmark of scleroderma; it occurs in 90–95 percent of patients. The remaining 5–10 percent usually have visceral involvement without skin involvement or Raynaud's phenomenon; this indicates that skin changes are not absolutely essential for the diagnosis.[12]

Skin involvement proceeds through three phases: edematous, indurative, and atrophic.[13] In the early *edematous phase,* there is painless, nonpitting, bilateral and symmetrical edema of the hands and fingers. The patient will experience a puffy and full feeling in the morning that improves during the day. On examination, nonpitting tautness is observed in the fingers, toes, and dorsal portions of the hands and feet. The face may also feel taut. In the *indurative phase,* edema is replaced by tight, hidebound skin that adheres to deeper structures (tendons, joints) and impedes their easy motion. The epidermis becomes thin, with loss of hair over affected areas. Although involvement of the hands is usually prominent and the most severe, any part of the body may be affected. In the *atrophic phase,* the skin becomes increasingly taut, thin, and shiny with marked loss of mobility. Contraction and hardening of the tissues leads to a loss of normal wrinkles and skin folds and to the development of a characteristic pinched, expressionless facies and hands drawn in fixed flexion (Fig. 3-1).

Commonly seen features include the following: flexion contractures of the hands and fingers, decrease in the maximum oral aperture, and skin hyperpigmentation, often stippled with spotty or patchy depigmentation that gives rise to a "salt-and-pepper" appearance; telangiectasias, chiefly on the fingers, palms, lips, and face; painful skin ulcerations, particularly over bony eminences, often secondarily infected chiefly by staphylococci; and subcutaneous calcification of the fingertips, extensor surfaces of the forearms, olecranon bursa, and prepatellar area.

At some time between 3 and 15 years after the appearance of classic skin changes, the hidebound dermis usually softens and becomes pliable; it may return to a near-normal stage.[2] This feature of the natural history of scleroderma has led to false enthusiasm for a variety of uncontrolled therapeutic trials. Insistence on controlled observations is the only safeguard to ensure valid conclusions. Control groups must be comparable to treated patients in the stage and degree of involvement with scleroderma.

A numerical skin-scoring system in which each interarticular area is graded from 0–4 (0 being normal and 4 hidebound skin) has been suggested to follow the progress of skin disease.[14] An association between high skin score and poor prognosis has been reported.[15]

The histologic appearance of involved skin varies, depending on the stage of cutaneous involvement (see the section on Pathogenesis). The weight of skin biopsies, obtained from the dorsum of the forearm and trimmed of all subcutaneous fat, is markedly greater than normal (mean 60 mg $\pm$ 1.3 SEM in scleroderma and 40.1 $\pm$ 0.9 mg in normal subjects).[13] Recently, using ultrasonic techniques, the mean dermal thickness in a group of scleroderma patients was measured at 7.7 mm, compared to 3.3 mm in control subjects.[16] This method may be of value in following the natural history or response to therapy in scleroderma. The remarkable reproducibility of control skin thickness implies careful regulation of this parameter. Skin thickness cannot

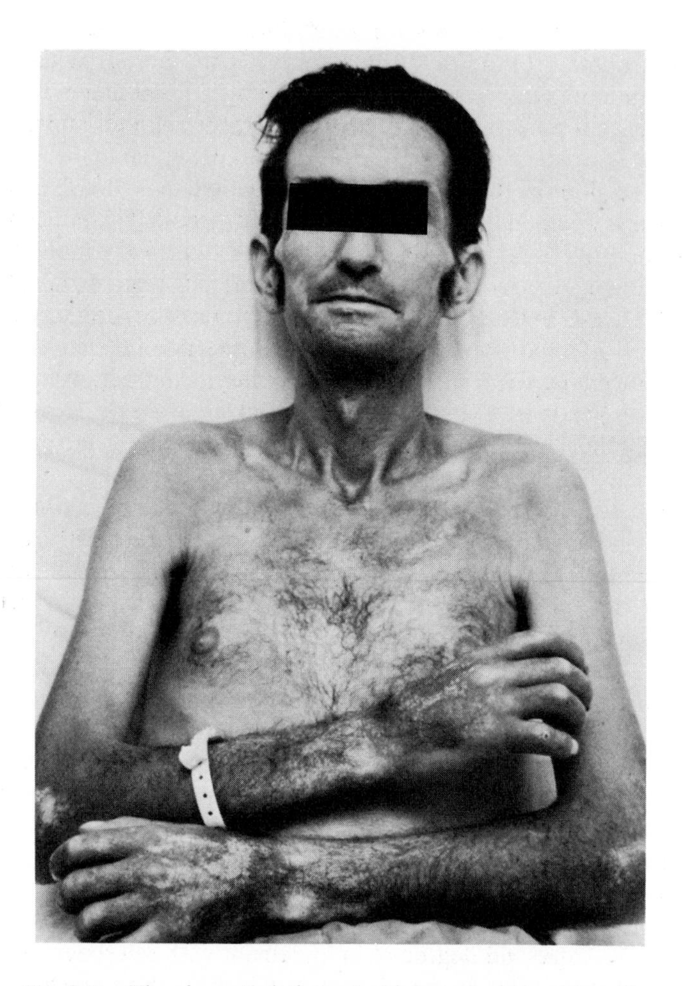

Fig. 3-1. The characteristic taut, thickened, shiny skin with pigmentary abnormalities of scleroderma. Hands show typical skin changes with flexion contractures and trophic ulcer.

distinguish between edema and fibrosis unless dry weight is also obtained. The natural history of dermal thickness should be further studied.

Muscles, Joints, and Bones

Arthralgias and joint stiffness are common in scleroderma and may be the presenting symptoms. True arthritis with warm or swollen joints is uncommon, but it does occur from the outset. In later stages of the disease, stiffness of the hands secondary to dermal involvement may be perceived as articular by the patient. Joint deformity usually results from fibrosis and contracture of skin rather than from articular disease per se. Sclerodermatous involvement of tendon sheaths can contribute to flexion contractures of joints. Examination may reveal audible or palpable crepitus over the tendon sheaths.

Radiographic studies rarely demonstrate erosive arthritis; indeed, bony erosions should suggest coexistent rheumatoid disease. A characteristic finding is resorption of the distal phalangeal tuft of fingers and toes. This is due to vascular disease and may be found in patients with severe Raynaud's phenomenon without scleroderma. Intra-articular calcium deposition with effusion has been reported. Pathologically, the synovium may show changes similar to, but less extensive than, those seen in rheumatoid arthritis: synovial proliferation and mononuclear cell infiltration. A distinctive finding is the deposition of a thick coat of fibrin over the synovium and, occasionally, within synovial tissue.

Disease of striated muscle is common in patients with scleroderma and may account for the frequent complaints of myalgia and weakness.[17] In general, however, muscle involvement is not severe. There may be muscle tenderness and objective weakness; more often, physical examination is unrevealing. Mild elevations of creatine phosphokinase and aldolase are seen in the majority of scleroderma patients. Electromyographic and histologic findings are usually normal but sometimes support the diagnosis of inflammatory myositis. Occasionally, myositis may dominate the clinical picture and result in severe proximal muscle weakness and tenderness, marked elevations in muscle enzymes, and grossly abnormal electromyograms. The term "sclerodermatomyositis" has been used to describe patients with cutaneous scleroderma and severe myositis.

Systemic Involvement.

Systemic involvement is of critical importance to prognosis and can be subtle in presentation.

Gastrointestinal Tract Involvement

This involvement is exceeded only by skin and joints in frequency of involvement. *Sjögren's syndrome* is seen in 20 percent of patients.[18] *Esophageal involvement* occurs in up to 80 percent; however, as many as 50 percent of these individuals remain asymptomatic.[19] Reduction in the propulsive force of the smooth muscle lining of the lower two-thirds of the esophagus is associated with gastroesophageal reflux. Dysphagia, a feeling of tightness under the sternum after eating, and occasional choking on food are common symptoms. The documentation of esophageal hypomotility by barium swallow or, more sensitively, by esophageal manometric studies supports the early diagnosis of scleroderma.[19] It is thus recommended that motility studies be done early in all patients. Cine-esophagram may detect complications of the scleroderma esophagus, such as gastric reflux and lower esophageal structure, while esophageal manometry is substantially more sensitive in detecting hypomotility.

Small Bowel Involvement

This is seen in as many as 50 percent of patients. Interestingly, it occurs almost exclusively in conjunction with esophageal disease. Occasionally duodenal–jejunal hypomotility is seen in the absence of skin involvement; this poses a diagnostic dilemma (systemic sclerosis sine scleroderma).[12] Symptoms are related to either intestinal stasis and/or malabsorption.[20] Abdominal distension, pain, nausea, and episodes of adynamic ileus may occur and mimic mechanical obstruction. Malabsorptive symptoms such as diarrhea and weight loss are seen in 10 percent of patients, particularly those with long-standing disease. Small bowel involvement can be best detected by standard upper gastrointestinal series showing dilatation and slow transit time and by 72 hour quantitative stool fat determinations following three days of a diet containing 100 gm of fat.

Large Bowel Involvement

Colonic disease is usually asymptomatic. Pseudo-obstruction, perforation, infarction, and hemorrhage are rarely seen, however. Radiographic studies reveal wide-mouth sacculation and dilatation. Decrease in colonic motility unresponsive to eating, neostigmine, or metaclopromide stimulation has been reported recently in a large proportion of patients.[21] Colonic involvement often parallels progression of the systemic disease.

Lung Involvement

Pulmonary involvement in scleroderma is of several types, which may exist separately or in combination: pleurisy, pulmonary hypertension with or without cor pulmonale, and diffuse interstitial lung disease. The most common pulmonary symptom is mild dyspnea on exertion and an intermittent cough which is occasionally productive of whitish sputum. The most frequent physical finding is the presence of dry, cracking inspiratory rales at the lung bases. An increased intensity of the pulmonic component of the second heart sound suggests pulmonary hypertension. With more advanced disease, this may be accompanied by fixed splitting of the second heart sound and findings of right ventricular hypertrophy.

The diffuse interstitial lung disease in scleroderma is due to a low-intensity alveolitis.[22] Unfortunately, early detection and precise techniques to evaluate alveolitis in scleroderma are not available. The gallium scan and pulmonary lavage have been advocated recently. Pulmonary function tests usually reveal impaired diffusion capacity and, occasionally, restricted vital capacity before any clinical or radiographic evidence of lung disease is present. Scleroderma lung disease usually does not lead to functional evidence of obstruction in peripheral airways; when the latter is found, it may be attributed to concomitant cigarette smoking.[23] The classic roentgenographic finding is interstitial markings most prominent at the lung bases. In early stages, an alveolar pattern may be present; this suggests an inflammatory component. A honeycomb pattern is a late manifestation. Pleural effusions are seen occasionally.

Pulmonary vascular involvement is common in scleroderma. Pulmonary vascular resistance has been reported to be increased in all patients studied by right-heart catheterization.[24] In approximately 50 percent of these patients, the increase in pulmonary vascular resistance was slight and did not produce clinical or radiographic signs of right ventrical hypertrophy. In the other patients, pulmonary hypertension was associated clinically with signs of right ventricular hypertrophy and histories of right ventricular failure. Interestingly, the pulmonary hypertension appeared to occur independently of alterations in pulmonary function or interstitial disease.

Severe pulmonary hypertension associated with advanced arteriolar lesions in the pulmonary arteries is seen in 25 percent of patients, some without apparent interstitial fibrosis.[25] The disease is characterized by progressive respiratory failure and severe pulmonary hypertension, this leads to death from a distinct clinicopathologic entity of malignant pulmonary hypertension, comparable to the better-recognized entity of malignant systemic hypertension in scleroderma. With the improved prognosis of renal scleroderma, pulmonary hypertension is an increasing cause of death in scleroderma.[26]

Lung abnormalities may not be due entirely to parenchymal lung disease. The known disturbances in esophageal motility may lead to aspiration pneumonia. Compression of the chest wall by tightened skin rarely affects respiratory function.

Cardiovascular Manifestations

Cardiac involvement may be subtle and relatively far advanced before it is recognized clinically. All three layers of the heart may be involved in scleroderma. Two clinical forms of pericardial disease can be seen in scleroderma[27]: chronic pericardial effusion, usually seen in association with dependent pitting edema, insidious dyspnea, Raynaud's phenomenon, cardiomegaly, congestive heart failure (with or without signs of tamponade), and pleural effusion. In 50 percent of patients with chronic pericardial effusion, renal failure developed within 6 months, an incidence severalfold higher than that expected in scleroderma without pericardial effusion. A separate clinical picture is more acute with pleuritic chest pain, dyspnea, pericardial friction rubs, fever, cardiomegaly, and elevated latex fixation titers. Pericardial disease is a relatively common form of cardiac involvement (62 percent incidence in autopsy studies), while echocardiographic evidence of pericardial effusion is seen in 20 percent of patients. Analysis of pericardial fluid reveals an exudative fluid with no evidence of autoantibodies, immune complexes, or complement depletion in contrast to pericardial fluids in rheumatoid arthritis or systemic lupus erythematosus.[28]

The true prevalence of myocardial and conduction system involvement is unknown. The onset of cardiac symptoms varies from insidious to fulminant. Sudden death, angina pectoris, and myocardial infarction have been seen in patients with scleroderma who have normal coronary arteries by angiography.[29] Arrhythmias are common with palpitation, syncope, and sudden death. Ventricular tachycardia may be the presenting symptom. In fact, cardiac disease preceded skin involvement in 3 of 9 and in 5 of 21 cases separately reported.[30,31] Physical examination may reveal cardiomegaly, gallop rhythm (S3 and S4), systolic murmur (usually poorly characterized), and diminished intensity of heart sounds. Edema may be difficult to appreciate due to hidebound skin. The major pathologic finding in the myocardium is fibrosis chronically and contraction band necrosis acutely; this results from intermittent interruption of circulation, an example of visceral Raynaud's phenomenon. Contraction band necrosis is a distinctive pathologic finding and appears to be the acute histopathologic manifestation of coronary reperfusion.[32] It can be produced in dogs by temporary coronary occlusion, and it is found in patients who died within 30 days of cardiac surgery. Histologic findings include transverse eosinophilic bands that represent condensation of contractile elements in myocardial cytoplasm between areas of increased granularity, abnormal location and appearance of mitochondria, dropout of nuclei, and paucity of inflammatory cells. Pathologic studies indicate progression from contraction band necrosis to myocardial fibrosis.

A prospective, noninvasive electrocardiographic study in scleroderma revealed abnormalities in 32 percent of patients on resting cardiogram, most commonly left anterior hemiblock and first degree heart block. The 24-hour electrocardiogram showed more serious abnormalities in 62 percent of the patients with supraventricular tachycardia, conduction disturbances (coupled ventricular extrasystoles), and ventricular tachycardia, which suggests more cardiac involvement than previously appreciated.[33] On echocardiogram, the following abnormalities are noted: increased left ventricular wall thickness, decreased left ventricular compliance, increased left atrial volume, diminished mitral valve closure velocity, and pericardial effusion.[34] Patchy decrease in myocardial uptake on thallium scintigraphic scan, or evidence of cold-induced myocardial dysfunction on thallium scan, or multiple-gaited acquisition radionuclide ventricular blood pool scan (MUGA) may improve the early detection of myocardial disease in scleroderma.

Involvement of the endocardium and heart valves has been reported but is uncommon and rarely causes functional abnormality. It should be remembered that pulmonary vascular disease, pericardial effusion, and systemic hypertension may lead to cardiac decompensation in scleroderma. Atherosclerosis and hypertensive heart disease are at least as common in scleroderma patients as they are in the general population of the same age and sex.

Renal involvement is the most common cause of death in scleroderma. Unfortunately, it may be sudden in onset with the occurrence of headache, blurred vision, hypertension with retinopathy and papilledema, oliguria, and sudden death.[35] Actually, the arterial proliferative lesion probably progresses in the kidney as in the other affected organs at a more or less constant pace throughout the course of the disease (Fig. 3-2). The sudden shutdown of renal cortical blood flow may be precipitated by a complex interaction of structural vascular disease, intravascular coagulation, and vasoconstriction with vessel damage via the renin–angiotensin–aldosterone pathway. It is important to identify patients with scleroderma who may develop renal involvement. At present, the best method of identification is to monitor all

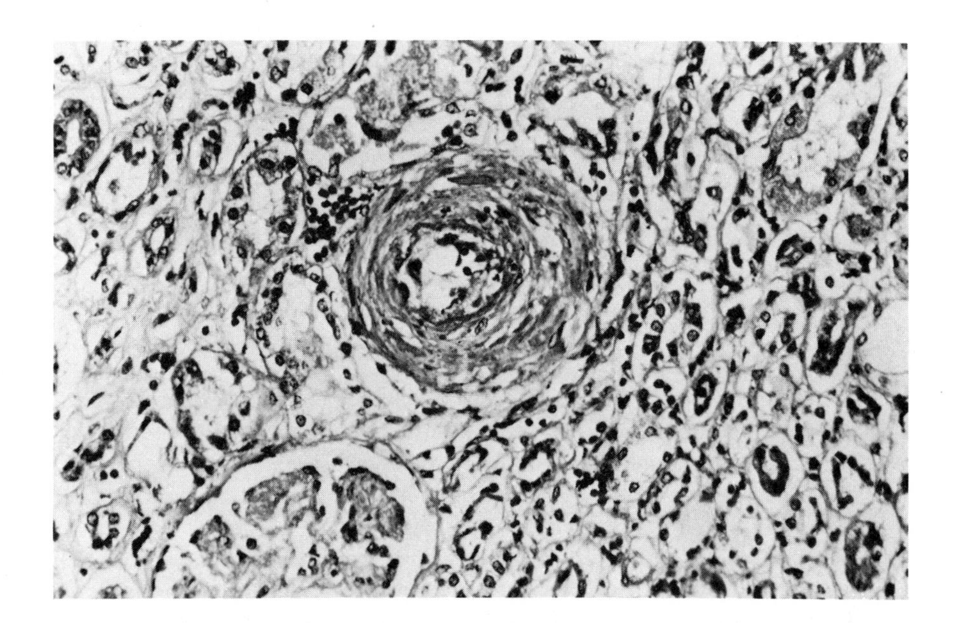

Fig. 3-2. Renal artery from the kidney of patient who died of oliguric renal failure with hypertension, which demonstrates the characteristic vascular lesion of scleroderma. This lesion shows intimal proliferation associated with fibrinoid necrosis and nuclear debris. H + E, X300. (From LeRoy EC: Scleroderma (systemic sclerosis), in Kelley WN, Harris ED Jr, Ruddy S, Sledge CB (eds): Textbook of Rheumatology. Philadelphia, W. B. Saunders, 1981. With permission.)

patients for proteinuria, azotemia, a change in baseline blood pressure level, microangiopathic hemolytic anemia, PAH clearance, and hyperreninemia.[36] The appearance of any abnormality of these features should lead to more intensive evaluation of renal blood flow by isotope clearance or angiography. The patient should be instructed in the self-determination of blood pressure and should perform it daily.

Thyroid Gland Involvement

Thyroid gland fibrosis and hypothyroidism, possibly of autoimmune pathogenesis, are frequent, although often unsuspected in scleroderma. Histologic evidence of severe fibrosis of the thyroid gland was found in 14 percent of scleroderma patients and in 2 percent of matched controls in autopsy studies. Some were clinically or chemically hypothyroid, particularly patients with limited cutaneous involvement of long standing.[37]

Neurologic Manifestations

Involvement of the nervous system in scleroderma is uncommon. Peripheral neuropathy has been reported but is rarely apparent clinically. Increased thickness of perineural connective tissue sheaths is seen histologically and may play a pathogenetic role. A number of patients with scleroderma have subsequently developed trigeminal neuralgia; involvement of other cranial nerves is rare. Similarly, central nervous system disease due to scleroderma is very rare, perhaps nonexistent.

PATHOGENESIS

General

The current pathogenetic hypothesis of scleroderma is based on immune–inflammatory events directed at the endothelium of the microvasculature, which leads to functional and structural vascular lesions that result in organ fibrosis (Fig. 3-3). Genetic predisposition and environmental factors have been suggested but are neither defined or definite.

The familial occurrence of scleroderma is usually regarded as rare.[38] It is of interest to note that close relatives of patients with scleroderma have been found to have low titers of ANAs and abnormally high frequency of chromosomal breakage. These two factors certainly lend support to the notion of familial predisposition to scleroderma. A variety of immunogenetic and epidemiologic studies have failed to support conclusively an association between HI-A antigens and scleroderma. Slightly increased frequencies of the HL-A antigens A9, Aw23 and Aw24, B8, B27 and B40, DRw4, DR5, DR2 and DR1 have been reported.[39,40,41]

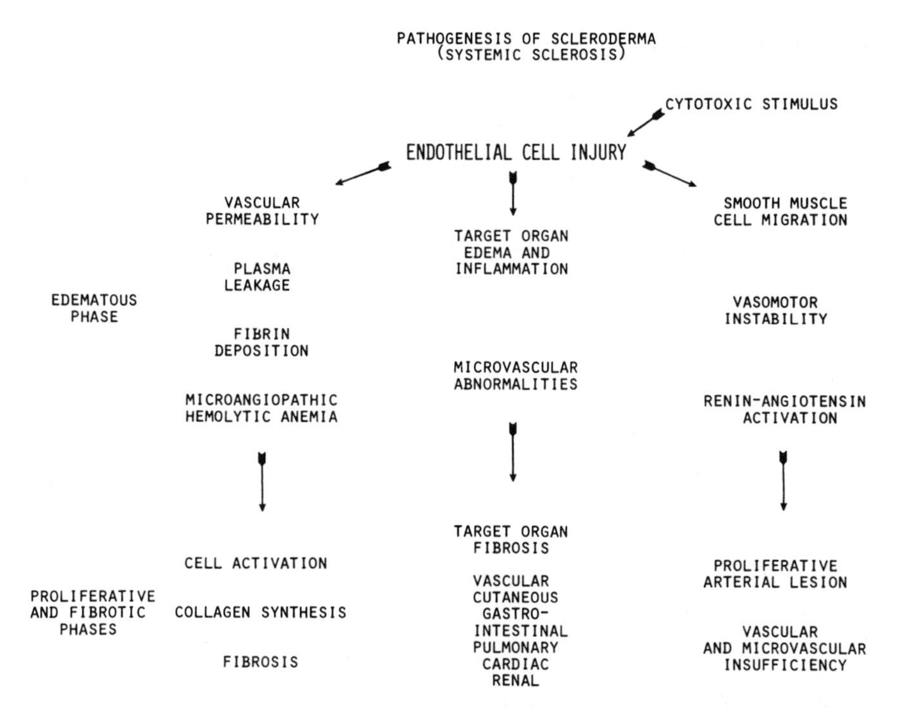

Fig. 3-3. Pathogenesis of scleroderma (systemic sclerosis). A working hypothesis concerning the pathogenetic features known or thought to play a role in scleroderma. (From LeRoy EC: Scleroderma (systemic sclerosis), in Kelley WN, Harris ED Jr, Ruddy S, Sledge CB (eds): Textbook of Rheumatology. Philadelphia. W. B. Saunders, 1981. With permission.)

Chromosomal abnormalities have been seen in 96 percent of patients with scleroderma.[42] The observed chromosomal abnormalities consist of chromatid-type aberration such as gaps and breaks of one or both chromatids and chromosome-type aberration such as acentric fragments, dicentrics, ring chromosomes derived from translocation or deletion of chromosome fragment, or intrachromosomal rearrangements. These abnormalities, which are acquired and therefore variable from cell to cell, are found in approximately 30 percent of mitotic cells. A similar proportion of abnormal cells has also been noted in asymptomatic siblings and family members of patients with scleroderma. A serum *breakage factor* has been noted in 37 of 42 scleroderma patients. Addition of this factor to lymphocyte cultures of healthy donors induced a threefold increase in chromosome and chromatid breaks. Unfortunately, little is known at this time about the nature of the breakage factor. Ultrafiltration studies, however, have shown that it is not a virus, thus negating the possibility of vertical transmission via a viral agent.[43] Indirect evidence suggests that oxygen-derived free radicals may be involved in the actual chromosome damage.

The Vascular Disorder in Scleroderma

The vascular features of scleroderma include Raynaud's phenomenon, an early edematous phase of the disorder, telangiectasias, capillary abnormalities as seen by nailfold and ultrastructural microscopy, and widespread vascular pathology noted in all involved organs.[44] The most striking histologic abnormalities occurs in small arteries and arterioles and consists of distinctive intimal proliferation of cells arranged concentrically in a matrix of ground substance. The cells are thought to originate from medial smooth muscle and to migrate toward the intima after injury to the endothelium. Evidence for endothelial injury includes the following: (1) absence of endothelium in association with thrombosis and fibrinoid necrosis on ultrastructural study of vascular lesions and (2) the duplication of endothelial basement membrane, a common observation in scleroderma known to occur after endothelial injury in other settings.

In certain instances, vascular lesions have been shown to antedate fibrosis. Many, if not all, clinical manifestations of scleroderma can be explained by functional and structural vascular compromise that follows repeated vascular injury, with subsequent healing of vascular wall and with proliferative vascular response and luminal narrowing. (Table 3-2) The coagulation cascade may be triggered by the intimal lesion that leads to fibrin deposits, reduced blood flow, and local ischemia Electron microscopic studies of skin biopsies from early stages have shown the presence of gaps between endothelial cells, as well as vacuolization and eventual destruction of endothelium. These changes are particularly marked in the upper dermis where endothelial cell remnants are occasionally seen obstructing the lumen.[45] Autoradiographic studies have shown a marked increase in endothelial labeling.[46] High endothelial cell labeling in vivo reflects endothelial damage; under normal in vivo conditions, the endothelial labeling index is estimated to be 0.4 percent or less. A labeling index of 2.4 percent was noted in scleroderma biopsies, while matched control biopsy showed less than 0.5 percent index. The mechanism of endothelial injury is not known; an endothelial specific cytotoxic factor in scleroderma sera has been observed in vitro.[47] The factor is a serine protease of unknown type, as cytotoxicity is abolished by soybean trypsin inhibitor and TLCK, a chloromethyl ketone inhibitor. Excess endogenous protease in scleroderma sera is demonstrated by the relative inability of scleroderma sera to inhibit tryptic hydrolysis of a synthetic substrate to the same degree as normal sera.[48] Experimental vascular studies have shown that intimal proliferation that follows endothelial injury is mediated by platelet interaction with the exposed subendothelium.[49] In vitro studies have shown that under normal conditions platelets do not interact with endothelial cells, while following endothelial injury "by hypotonic treatment," intense platelet adhesion is seen.[50]

Factor VIII–von Willebrand factor attachment to subendothelium has been shown to be an important step in the first phase of platelet interaction

Table 3-2
Probable Mechanism of Drug Therapy as Related to Pathogenesis of Scleroderma

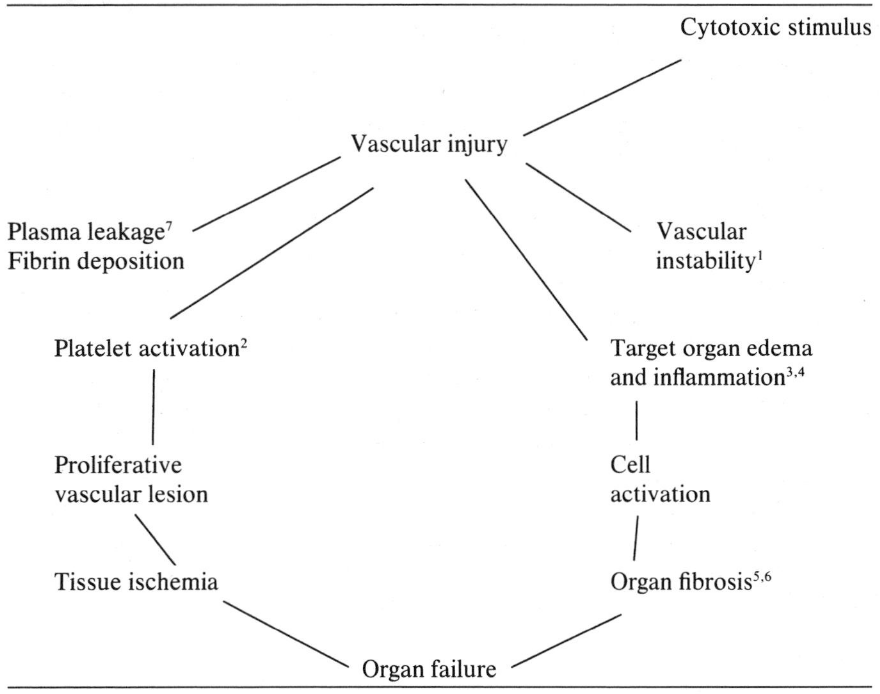

1, Vasodilators; 2, Antiplatelet Agents; 3, Glucocorticoids; 4, Immunosuppressive agents,; 5, D-penicillamine; 6, Colchicine; 7, Anabolic steroids

with the vascular wall. Once endothelial cells are injured, von Willebrand factor binds to the subendothelium and mediates platelet adhesion.[51]

Von Willebrand factor activity and factor VIII–von Willebrand factor antigen concentration were significantly elevated in patients with scleroderma.[52] The observed increases may be due to endothelial injury, since subjecting endothelial cells to various forms of injury in vitro results in a marked increase in von Willebrand factor activity.[52] In experimental animal studies, acute endothelial injury of the pulmonary microcirculation led to marked increases in circulating von Willebrand factor levels[53]; furthermore, in experimental atherosclerosis, studies have implicated von Willebrand factor in the development of the proliferative vascular lesion, since both naturally occurring and diet-induced atherosclerosis do not develop to the same extent in von Willebrand factor-deficient swine compared to swine with normal von Willebrand factor levels.[54] Whether the increased levels seen in scleroderma enhance the development of structural vascular lesion or merely reflects the extent of endothelial injury remains to be resolved. Von Willebrand factor levels in scleroderma patients have been shown to increase further after cold exposure; this underscores the need for strict prevention of vasospasm (Raynaud's phenomenon), which may contribute significantly to the perpetuation of the vascular disease in scleroderma.[52]

Following platelet adhesion, platelet aggregation and release of platelet granule contents is seen (Tables 3-3 and 3-4). Both the rate of platelet adherance to exposed subendothelium and the degree of intimal proliferation are direct consequences of endothelial loss from the luminal vascular surface.[55] Formed platelet aggregates persist by continuous dynamic aggregation and deaggregation with eventual phagocytosis by the reticuloendothelial system. The number of circulating platelet aggregates has been shown to correlate significantly with platelet survival time—the more aggregates, the shorter the platelet half-life. An increase in circulating platelet aggregates has been reported in scleroderma.[56] Secreted platelet proteins have various biologic functions; these include procoagulant, antiheparin, and growth promoting activities.[57] Some of these proteins, such as platelet factor IV and β-thromboglobulin, are found only in platelets, and hence, serve as markers of platelet release. Plasma concentrations of each is a reliable index of platelet consumption in vivo. In the absence of renal failure or immune thrombocytopenia, plasma β-thromboglobulin levels correlate with platelet survival as measured by chromium platelet survival time.[58] Increases in the plasma level of β-thromboglobulin have been reported in scleroderma.[56] The biologic function of β-

Table 3-3
Secreted Platelet Granule Proteins

Secreted Platelet Granule Proteins
Platelet specific proteins
Platelet factor 4
β-thromboglobulin
Platelet derived growth factor
Vascular permeability factor
Bacteriocidal and chemotactic factor
Enzymes
Cathepsins
β-galactosidase
Neutral protease
Cyclic -3, 5′-phosphodiesterase
Plasma proteins
Albumin, fibrinogen
Factor V, VIII
α_1-antitrypsin
α_2-macroglobulin
Fibronectin
Antiplasmin
Inhibitors of plasminogen activator

thromboglobulin is not known, but recent studies suggest that it reduces the production of prostacyclin in cultured bovine endothelial cells, which possess a specific receptor for β-thromboglobulin.[59] The characteristics of this receptor would permit β-thromboglobulin to act locally at high concentrations to favor platelet aggregation by diminishing prostacyclin production. Several factors govern platelet interaction with the vascular wall, including endothelial injury, the rate and character of blood flow, the concentration of von Willebrand factor, and the prostacyclin/thromboxane ratio in the vascular microenvironment. In scleroderma, most of these mechanisms have been shown to be operative. In vivo platelet adhesion to subendothelium in scleroderma has been reported and was found to precede the development of proliferative vascular lesions.[60] Furthermore, the predominant site of vascular disease in scleroderma is the small arteriole and the microcirculation where the flow is more steady and less pulsatile; these are conditions that enhance platelet adherence to subendothelium compared to large arteries and pulsatile flow.[61]

Intimal vascular proliferation may lead to activation of the coagulation cascade. Studies of fibrinogen half-life revealed rapid fibrinogen turnover in scleroderma.[62] Patients with "rapidly progressive" disease had a more rapid fibrinogen disappearance than did those with "stable" disease. The mean fibrinogen half-life of 8 patients given intravenous heparin increased significantly; this suggested that fibrinogen in these patients was capable of normal survival and that an increase in fibrinogen consumption and turnover is common in scleroderma. An occasional patient with major arterial and venous thrombosis is consistent with a hypercoagulable state in scleroderma.[63] Impaired fibrinolysis as measured by the euglobulin clot lysis time is common in scleroderma and is probably due to defective synthesis, storage, or release of plasminogen activator from the vascular endothelium.[64] Raynaud's phenomenon may also contribute since fibrinolytic activity of normal skin flaps subjected to ischemia and reperfusion revealed marked decrease in fibrinolytic activity in reperfused tissue.[65] Fibrin deposition in vivo may trigger endothelial contraction; this leads to platelet adherence to the vessel wall in the presence of inadequate fibrinolysis,[66] which eventually results in prolif-

Table 3-4
Alteration of Platelet Parameters in Scleroderma

Alteration of Platelet Parameters in Scleroderma
Increased platelet aggregate ratio
Increased plasma levels of
β-thromboglobulin
platelet factor 4
Increased surface activation
Increased in vitro aggregability

erative vascular lesions. This view highlights reduced fibrinolytic activity and enhanced fibrinogen consumption in the evolution of the proliferative vascular disorder; both defects have been observed in scleroderma.

The proliferative-occlusive vascular lesions lead to underperfusion of involved organs, as shown by decreased skin blood flow when measured by clearance of radioactive xenon. Increase in blood flow has been demonstrated following administration of guanethidine,[67] PGE_1,[68] PGI_2,[69] and the anabolic steroid stanozolol,[70] this indicates the partial reversibility of the vascular disease. The capacity of blood vessels to reendothelialize has been shown in other settings. Until the mechanisms of vascular damage in scleroderma are fully understood, therapeutic intervention may lack a rational basis. Until this time, however, attempts to interrupt the cycle of endothelial injury, platelet adherance and release, intravascular coagulation, and defective fibrinolysis seem warranted if risks are acceptable.

Fibrosis

A growing body of evidence now suggests that the increase in collagenous connective tissue in scleroderma patients is the result of augmented collagen synthesis by fibroblasts (Tables 3-5 and 3-6).[71] Histological studies of early skin lesions in scleroderma revealed increased numbers of fibroblasts. The cells have well-developed rough endoplasmic reticulum "suggestive of active collagen synthesis"; also fine collagen fibrils (100Å–400Å) that represent "young collagen" are found around the cells. Deposition of type III collagen in the dermis "particularly the lower dermis" is seen in the early stages of scleroderma.[72] Later, in the fibrotic stage, dense collagen, which consists almost exclusively of type I collagen, is seen.

Immunofluorescence studies, semiquantitative at best, suggest increased levels of type III collagen, as well as type I and type IV, in cultures from deep dermal biopsies of patients with scleroderma.[73] Biochemical studies of fibroblasts in culture, however, showed the normal proportions (20 percent) of type III collagen synthesized.[74] These studies are not necessarily contradictory but may reflect the general situation in which type III collagen is synthesized early in all inflammatory reactions and in which type I collagen is predominant in all human fibrotic reactions in later stages.

Fibroblast cultures established by explant culture of dermis from scleroderma patients have shown increased collagen accumulation. Cultures from lower dermis accumulated more collagen than those from upper dermis. Enhanced collagen accumulation in fibroblast culture has been shown to be caused by increased collagen synthesis per cell. Furthermore, enhanced collagen accumulation persists for many generations in culture; this suggests that disordered regulation of connective tissue synthesis or degradation by the fibroblast is of importance in the pathogenesis of scleroderma.[75]

Table 3-5
Chain, Molecular Composition, and Tissue Distribution of Collagen Types

Type	Chain	Molecular form	Distribution
I	$\alpha_1(I)$	$[\alpha_1(I)]_2\alpha 2$	Bone, dermis, tendon
	α_2	$[\alpha_1(I)]_3$	arterial wall, dentin
II	$\alpha_1(II)$	$[\alpha_1(II)]_3$	Hyaline cartilages
III	$\alpha_1(III)$	$[\alpha_1(III)]_3$	Arterial wall, dermis uterine wall
IV	α_1,α_2	Not established	Basement membrane
V	$\alpha_1,\alpha_2,\alpha_3$	Not established	Link basement membrane to stroma

A consistent and reproducible manifestation of the fibrotic potential of scleroderma is the demonstration that scleroderma dermal fibroblasts in vitro differ from control fibroblasts in several characteristics: (1) scleroderma fibroblasts produce several times more collagen per cell, (2) scleroderma fibroblasts are less sensitive to the mitogenic stimuli of serum than are control fibroblasts, and (3) other connective tissue components (fibronectin and proteoglycans) are synthesized at increased levels by scleroderma fibroblasts.

Collagen is synthesized in a precursor form, which contains at both ends globular extensions. These extensions are cleaved by procollagen peptidases. The amino terminal procollagen peptides can inhibit the production of α-1 and α-2 chain synthesis. Radiolabeled procollagen peptides are taken up by fibroblasts and are deposited near the rough endoplasmic reticulum, presumably at the site of protein synthesis. Recent data indicate that the peptides lead to a specific inhibition of translation of collagen mRNA, while translation of other mRNAs is not affected.[76] These same propeptides also reduce the enhanced collagen synthesis of scleroderma skin fibroblast in culture; this demonstrates the capacity of scleroderma cells to be regulated at least by

Table 3-6
The Fibrotic Potential of Scleroderma Fibroblasts

Increased collagen synthesis
Increased proteoglycans and fibronectin synthesis
Possible decreased collagenase synthesis
Insensitivity to mitogenic stimulus
Tolerance to "starvation environment"

collagen propeptides. The inhibition of collagen synthesis by amino-terminal type I peptides applies to both types I and III collagens and, in that sense, is nonspecific.

Initial studies of dermal fibroblasts assumed that skin is a homogenous organ whose interstitial cells react similarly. More recent studies of both healthy and scleroderma skin, however, have noted differences between upper (papillary) and lower (reticular) dermal cells. In healthy skin, papillary fibroblasts show greater proliferative capacity, both by more rapid population doublings and by more population doublings before termination of growth. In scleroderma cells, increased levels of collagen synthesis are seen largely in cultures of lower or reticular dermal fibroblasts. Immunofluorescent analysis of skin biopsies from scleroderma patients with specific antibodies against interstitial collagens and procollagens, against fibronectin and, against the basement membrane proteins type IV collagen and laminin revealed distinctly increased staining for type I procollagen and fibronectin in the lower dermis and subcutaneous tissue when compared with normal skin; this suggests that fibrosis begins around capillaries and in close proximity to adipose tissue. The distribution of type IV collagen and laminin was altered in some patients, which probably reflects differences in small blood vessels.[77]

Currently, two hypotheses attempt to explain the abnormal behavior of scleroderma fibroblasts in vitro: One proposes "fibroblast activation" and alteration in the regulation of collagen synthesis at the cellular level. The second indicates that normal dermal fibroblasts are heterogeneous with respect to levels of collagen synthesis, and scleroderma fibroblasts are subject to a selection process that favors the growth of high-collagen-producing cell. These hypotheses are not mutually exclusive since selection could also involve activation of collagen synthesis. A recent study[78] of human skin fibroblasts cloned in vitro showed threefold difference in collagen synthesis in 21 clones from a single biopsy of healthy newborn skin; this heterogeneity of phenotypic expression was observed over multiple population doublings. When the clones were exposed to sera from 10 scleroderma patients, selective growth of high-collagen-producing clones was observed; the same clones showed an insensitivity to feeding schedules similar to fibroblasts from scleroderma skin. These data raise the possibility that scleroderma represents a process of selection of fibroblasts programmed to produce increased amounts of collagen.

The in vivo mitogenic factor, which could both select and activate, may well be the recently described mitogenic activity in scleroderma sera. The factor induced significant increases in control fibroblast numbers. The effect was abrogated by protease inhibitors (soybean trypsin inhibitor and TLCK). The biological role of this activity is not yet defined.[79]

In addition to enhanced collagen synthesis by scleroderma fibroblasts, a decrease in collagenase synthesis has been reported[80]; other studies failed to confirm that finding.[81] The control mechanisms of collagenase synthesis and release are not known. Several different cell types produce collagenase in a latent form, which can be activated by plasmin and perhaps other proteinases. Macrophages have been shown to release a plasminogen activator; moreover, coculture of peripheral blood monocytes and fibroblasts leads to enhanced synthesis and release of collagenase by fibroblasts.[82] Better understanding of collagen degradation in scleroderma is needed. The regulation of fibroblast proliferation and connective tissue synthesis in health and in disease is poorly understood. The study of scleroderma may lead to a better understanding of fibrotic disorders in general.

The Immune–Inflammatory Process

Although a variety of immunologic abnormalities has been described in scleroderma, most are low level and usually nondiagnostic. Patients with scleroderma have an increased risk to develop autoimmune disorders; conversely, patients with systemic lupus erythematosus and other connective tissue disorders often have a variety of scleroderma-like features.

Humoral Immune Phenomena

Hypergammaglobulinemia is a frequent finding in patients with scleroderma.[83] No consistent abnormality of specific serum immunoglobulin classes or subclasses has been found, however, ANAs are common findings in sera of patients; however, the frequency of detection varies greatly among investigators. ANAs have been detected in sera from 33 to 96 percent of patients. (Table 3-7) This discrepancy is most likely due to the particular substrate used in the indirect immunofluorescence procedure. Using cultured human laryngeal-cell carcinoma cells (HEP_2), ANAs were found in 96 percent of patients.[84] In a small proportion of patient sera, antigenic specificity to SCL-70 (nonhistone nuclear protein, 70,000 daltons), 4–6S nuclear RNA, and

Table 3-7
Autoantibodies in Scleroderma (Frequency, %)

ANA	33–96
Anti-centromeric	57
Anti-Scl-70	18
Anti-RNA	100
Anti-RNP	21
Anti-α-globulin	22–50
Anti-thyroid	16
Anti-type I Collagen	86
Anti-type V Collagen	54
Anti-fibroblasts	70

nuclear ribonucleoprotein (RNP) have been observed.[85] Antibody to SCL-70 antigen is relatively specific for scleroderma but seen in only 20–25 percent of patient sera.[84] This antibody specificity has not been found in SLE or RA, although it has been found on occasion in patients with Raynaud's disease or Sjögren's syndrome. Antibodies to RNA in scleroderma are often directed to uracil and specific for ss-RNA. Anti-RNA antibodies found in SLE differ in their specificity compared to those in scleroderma. SLE sera react with poly-A and poly-U; this indicates recognition of helical structure in double-stranded RNA; in scleroderma, antibodies react with poly-U but not with poly-A, which suggests base-specific rather than helix-specific reactivity.[86] No relationship has been found between the duration or severity of disease and the presence of levels or types of ANA.

Ninety-eight percent of the sera from patients with limited cutaneous scleroderma (CREST syndrome) contain high titers of antibodies that produces a discrete, speckled pattern of immunofluorescence on human laryngeal carcinoma cells (HEP_2). The antibody has been shown to react with the centromeric region of metaphase chromosomes.[87] These antibodies have also been found in 3 of 14 patients with Raynaud's disease, in 1 of 60 patients with SLE, in 3 of 26 patients with diffuse scleroderma, and in 1 of 15 patients with mixed or overlap connective tissue syndromes. Anticentromere antibodies were not detected in the serum of patients with rheumatoid arthritis, sicca syndrome, or linear scleroderma. Antibodies to cell surface membrane of viable fibroblasts were found in 70 percent of patients with scleroderma.[88] Antibodies to type I and type IV collagens were detected in the sera of patients with scleroderma.[89] Antibodies to type IV collagen correlated with the presence of abnormal pulmonary diffusion capacity. Antibody responses to autologous collagens may lead to a self-perpetuating cycle: complement activation, immune complex formation, and antibody-dependent cell-mediated cytotoxity.

Cell-Mediated Immune Observations

Mononuclear cell infiltrates are frequently seen in scleroderma, particularly in the perivascular region. Electron microscopic studies have identified the presence of mature lymphocytes, T lymphoblasts, immature plasma cells, plasma cells, and macrophages in early subcutaneous lesions.[90] In the fibrotic stage, fibroblasts and histiocytes predominate. The presence of T and B cells in early lesions suggests that both cellular and humoral immunity participate in the pathogenesis of scleroderma. Most of these cells are seen around capillaries; T cells can be seen migrating through endothelial cell gaps. The presence of monocytes suggests activation of T cells with possible release of monocyte-derived chemotactic migration inhibitors.

Studies of T-cell subpopulations and immunoregulatory networks in scleroderma have revealed normal postthymic precursors (autologous rosette-forming T cells), normal concanavalin-induced suppressor cells, normal spontaneously expanded precursor cell function, and decreased circulating T-gamma cells (roughly speaking, T gamma cells are helper cells); however, helper function is not only intact but also is significantly increased.[91] The reduced number may be due to redistribution of cells into the extravascular space, or the presence of lymphocytotoxic antibody, or decreased generation. Increased helper function could result in both an increase in B-cell function with autoantibody production and in production of lymphokines.

Impairment of lymphocyte transformation responses to phytohemagglutinin correlated well with both the number of circulating T lymphocytes and the extent of visceral involvement.[92] Furthermore, sera from patients with scleroderma induced suppression of lymphocyte transformation when added to cultures of normal lymphocytes.

Antibody-dependent cell-mediated cytotoxicity (ADCC) that involves peripheral blood mononuclear cells in scleroderma is selectively decreased against Chang liver cells, which may indicate reduction in the effector cell population similar to findings in SLE.[93]

The recent development of heterologus monoclonal antibodies has enabled more comprehensive quantification of T-cell subpopulations. A subset of scleroderma patients (30 percent) exhibits an elevated ratio of OKT4/OKT8 cells, which could be accounted for mainly be reduction in OKT8 cells compared with controls.[94] This numerical imbalance in lymphocyte subpopulations may be widespread in autoimmune diseases. Antigen-specific suppressor-cell activity has been shown to be normal in scleroderma patients.

Peripheral blood lymphocytes from patients with scleroderma were found to be cytotoxic to cultures of fibroblasts, epithelial and muscle cells of skin, renal and muscle origin; these findings were independent of the severity of the clinical condition, including the presence or absence of myopathy.[95]

The role of inflammatory cells in vascular pathology and tissue fibrosis has been studied recently. Perivascular infiltration of lymphocyte and monocytemacrophages are responsible for destruction of the microvasculature in the first set skin-graft rejection. In scleroderma, mononuclear cell infiltration precedes vascular degeneration, fibroblast proliferation, and collagen deposition.

Cell-mediated immunity to skin extract and collagen has been observed in scleroderma.[96] Sixty-two percent of patients with diffuse scleroderma responded to soluble extracts of both normal and scleroderma skin in the macrophage-migration inhibition test. Furthermore, studies on cutaneous extracts have identified the active antigen to be a low molecular weight substance (approximately 3,500 dalton) that contains RNA-polypeptides.[97]

Cell-mediated immunity to collagen and other skin components could maintain inflammation, recruit monocytes that participate in microvascular destruction, and stimulate collagen synthesis. The hypothesis that immunologically mediated inflammation with monocyte participation is important in scleroderma is strengthened by the high incidence of scleroderma-like lesions in patients undergoing chronic graft versus host reaction following bone marrow transplantation.[98] A granulomatous response to foreign material may also lead to a scleroderma-like disorder in patients with augmentation mammaplasty.[99]

The hypothesis would suggest that altered endothelial antigens (neoantigens) trigger cell-mediated immunity, which would initiate and maintain a monocyte inflammatory response. Monocyte activation releases factors that damage endothelium and diffuse to the interstitium to activate fibroblasts. The presence of perivascular cellular infiltrates in scleroderma is consistent with this view. Furthermore, supernatant fluid of normal human peripheral blood mononuclear cell culture has been shown to stimulate human dermal fibroblast growth and to suppress endothelial cell growth in vitro.[100] The soluble factor or factors were shown to be released by the phagocytic population of peripheral blood mononuclear cells, were nondialyzable, and were rapidly released by the cells in vitro, which were detectable at 2 hours and reach plateau levels by 24 hours. The same factor has been shown to be released by scleroderma monocytes. The activity is blocked by protease inhibitors (TLCK, PMSF, and soybean trypsin inhibitor).[101] The activity may be identical to that recently described from macrophages obtained by bronchoalveolar lavage.[102] A fibroblast growth-promoting activity (molecular weight, 18,000 daltons) appeared to be distinct from other characterized growth factors. The alveolar macrophage-derived growth factor stimulated lung fibroblast DNA synthesis within 12 hours, with cell division apparent within 48 hours. In serum-free culture, the alveolar-derived growth factor by itself did not promote fibroblast replication but rather acted as a progression factor, which causes a synergistic increase in fibroblast replication rate in the presence of competence factors such as fibroblast growth factor or platelet-derived growth factor.

Inflammatory lesions are characterized by participation and interaction of several different cell types. One example is the cooperation of lymphocytes and monocytes in immune responses, an interaction mediated in part by the release of soluble factors (lymphokines and monokines), which affect cell metabolism. The relationship between mononuclear cells and other cell types in inflammation is less well defined. Despite the substantial number of immune network irregularities that have been described in scleroderma, none as yet has uniquely distinguished scleroderma from other diffuse connective tissue disorders nor explained the virtually unique capacity of scleroderma patients for extensive fibrosis.

DIFFERENTIAL DIAGNOSIS

The differential diagnosis of scleroderma includes rare conditions that may mimic the cutaneous manifestation but are distinguished, by the lack of the classic visceral involvement and by their own characteristic clinical features.

Eosinophilic Fasciitis

This is a recently described syndrome[103] characterized by inflammation and thickness of the fascia with skin induration (resembling scleroderma) and eosinophilia. The age of onset ranges from 4 to 88 years of age and the disease appears to be more prevalent in males. The onset may be preceded by trauma or unusually strenuous physical exertion and is characterized by painful swelling and induration of the skin of the forearms and legs and the proximal portions of the extremities, the trunk, and the neck. The skin surface has a cobblestone appearance. Raynaud's phenomenon and the internal manifestation of scleroderma are conspicuously absent. Characteristically, eosinophilia is present in the early stages and hypergammaglobulinemia is common. Histologic diagnosis is established by means of full-thickness biopsy that includes skin, subcutaneous tissue, fascia, and muscle. Inflammation and fibrosis are found in the fascia, which may be thickened many times more than normal. A large number of lymphocytes, plasma cells, eosinophils, and histocytes are present in the affected tissue. Corticosteroids in small doses usually provide substantial relief. Aplastic anemia and/or thrombocytopenic purpura have been reported in a small number of patients whose skin disease is in clinical remission.

Scleredema

Scleredema is a connective tissue disease characterized by sudden, rapidly progressive induration of the skin.[104] In approximately two-thirds of patients skin induration is preceded by an infectious process, usually pharyngitis of streptococcal origin. There is a high frequency of diabetes mellitus in adults with scleredema. The disease manifests as a progressive, painless, symmetrical edematous induration of the skin of face, scalp, neck, trunk, and proximal portions of the extremities. The hands and feet are spared. Histochemical examination of the skin reveals dense deposits of mucopolysaccharide, mainly hyaluronic acid. The disease tends to resolve after a period of 6–12 months, but in children it may persist in a mild degree for many years. It may persist indefinitely in patients with diabetes mellitus. There is no known effective treatment for scleredema.

Vinyl Chloride Disease

A high incidence of scleroderma-like illness has been described in workers involved in the process of polymerization of polyvinyl chloride.[105] This syndrome, also known as acro-osteolysis, may occur after years of exposure to the chemical. The clinical picture includes Raynaud's phenomenon, induration of the skin of the hands and forearms, and osteolytic and sclerotic lesions of the bones, particularly of the distal phalanges. A high incidence of hepatic angiosarcoma superimposed on hepatic fibrosis has been reported.

Bleomycin-Induced Fibrosis

Administration of the tumoricidal drug bleomycin leads to the development of collagenous plaques or nodules in the skin.[106] Other cutaneous manifestations consist of linear hyperpigmentation, alopecia, nail changes, and gangrene of the digits that simulates scleroderma. A fibrotic process similar to the one seen in the skin may take place in the lung, which usually affects the lower lobes. This process may be progressive and fatal.

Pentazocine-Induced Fibrosis

Flat or nodular sclerosis of the dermis at the site of injection of pentazocine has been reported.[107] Fibrosis of underlying muscle gives rise to contractures. Histologic examination of affected tissue reveals fibrosis of the dermis and subcutaneous tissue and fibrous myopathy.

Scleromyxedema

This is a rare disorder in which there is a widespread lichenoid eruption of soft, small, pale red or yellowish papules in association with diffuse skin thickening, which includes the face and hands.[108] Acid mucopolysaccharides are found between collagen bundles on biopsy. Abnormal serum immunoglobulins (M component) are often present; this suggests a relationship between this condition and plasma cell dyscrasias.

Porphyria Cutanea Tarda

This is a relatively rare disease characterized by an abnormality in pyrrole metabolism.[104] The disease may be associated with scleroderma-like changes that resemble morphea, linear scleroderma, or generalized scleroderma. Skin induration often starts on exposed areas, i.e., face, V area of the neck and chest. On biopsy, increased collagen in the dermis and deposits of IgG and IgM around blood vessels and at the epidermal–dermal junction in sun-exposed area have been noted.

Carcinoid syndrome

Sclerosis of the skin on the legs has been described in a few patients with the carcinoid syndrome.[109] Skin biopsy reveals dense collagen bundles and mononuclear cell infiltrates. It has been suggested that serotonin may be responsible for the fibrosis of the lung and skin in this syndrome. Functioning carcinoid tumors release large amounts of serotonin, which causes a syndrome characterized by dyspnea, cough and wheezing, diarrhea, and fibrosis of the pulmonary and tricuspid valves and the inferior vena cava.

Chronic Graft-versus-Host Disease

Allogeneic bone marrow transplantation may lead to a graft-versus-host reaction, which results in a syndrome characterized by skin rash, hepatitis, diarrhea, and lymphopenia. The cutaneous manifestations of the chronic graft-versus-host disease include hyperpigmentation, scleroderma-like lesions that are usually preceded by maculopapular rash, and a measles-like exanthem.[98] Biopsies of scleroderma-like lesions have revealed lymphocytic infiltration of the basal cell layers around blood vessels, vacuolization of basal cells, and fibrosis of the dermis and subcutaneous tissue. Sjögren's syndrome has been reported in most patients with chronic graft-versus-host disease. The association of scleroderma-like lesions, Sjögren's syndrome, and graft-versus-host disease is probably more than fortuitous and strongly suggests that activation of immune networks play a role in the pathogenesis of scleroderma. Chronic graft-versus-host disease represents a widespread activation of the immune system; the leading question is which aspect of immune activation promotes the vascular and fibrotic reactions *not* seen in other types of immune disorders.

Other rare conditions that could mimic scleroderma skin disease include progeria (Werner's syndrome), phenylketonuria, and primary amyloidosis.

TREATMENT

Since no single therapeutic modality has been shown to improve all the manifestations of scleroderma, an approach directed at both the pathophysiologic and the clinical expression of the disease is recommended. The general management plan includes supportive measures, use of drugs that are potentially efficacious, and management of individual organ involvement. (Table 3-2)

1. Supportive Measures. These consist of patient and family counseling, avoidance of exposure to cold and trauma, and the use of physical therapy. Frequently, the psychologic aspects of chronic disease are given inadequate attention by the physician. It is essential to encourage the patient to lead as normal a life as possible, within the limitations created by the disease. Physical activity should be encouraged; early discussion of how the disorder may change the patient's family, occupational, and social life can foster gradual emotional adjustment to such changes. Continuing emotional support is a major component in the overall management of scleroderma. The physician should discuss with the patient and his or her family the alterations in appearance brought about by scleroderma. In most patients scleroderma will impose a major change in life style. Physical therapy is an important adjunct in the management and should include active and passive range-of-motion exercises and heat

to improve circulatory flow and impede contractions caused by fibrotic skin and joints. It is important to maintain maximum function during the active phase of the disease so that when activity subsides, the patient will be in an optimally functional state. The use of massage and heat (molten paraffin, warm whirlpool, and hot water baths) and traction splints may be necessary to reduce the rate of progression of contractures. Liberal application of petroleum or lanolin lubricant helps protect the skin during active exercise.

2. Drug Therapy. The mainstays of drug therapy include antiplatelet drugs, vasodilators, corticosteroids, D-penicillamine, and colchicine.

Antiplatelet Therapy

In general, the use of antiplatelet agents assumes that platelet activation (adhesion, aggregation, and release) plays an important role in initiation or perpetuation of the vascular disease in scleroderma. In recent years, interest in platelet involvement in the scleroderma vascular lesions has emerged, and evidence for intense interaction of platelets with the vessel wall has been presented *(videsupra)*. The clinical use of antiplatelet therapy should always be monitored with appropriate parameters of in vivo (rather than in vitro) platelet activation. Aspirin (150 mg every 3 days or 40 mg once daily) has been shown to inhibit the generation of the vasoconstricting and platelet-aggregating thromboxane A_2 but not the vasodilating and platelet-disaggregating prostaglandin I_2 Dipyridamole (200–400 mg daily in divided doses) diminishes platelet adherence to damaged vessels by increasing platelet cyclic adenosine 5′-monophosphate levels and by stimulating prostaglandin I_2 release from the vascular endothelium. Dipyridamole also inhibits adenosine uptake by endothelial cells; this enhances adenosine concentrations locally, which is vasodilatory. Another approach is the use of continuous intravenous infusions of prostaglandin I_2 at doses of from 2 to 20 ng/kg/min for 3 days. This therapy produces striking and prolonged clinical improvement in digital ulceration and the frequency and severity of Raynaud's phenomenon.[69] This approach opens a new era in the pharmacologic therapy of scleroderma. Preliminary results are encouraging; the long-term effect on either the mortality rate or the incidence of organ failure is unknown.

Vasodilators and Sympatholytic Agents

These agents are indicated for prevention of Raynaud's attacks, particularly when ulcers, digital infarcts, gangrene, and persistent and infected paronychia are present. Even without these complications, the use of these drugs in stable patients is justified, since Raynaud's phenomenon in the involved viscera may contribute significantly to the pathogenesis *(vide supra)*. The following agents have been used with equal success: nitroglycerin, applied topically directly to digits, 2 or 3 times daily; griseofulvin, 125–150 mg twice a day; tolazoline, 80 mg twice a day; reserpine, 0.25–0.50 mg daily; α-methyldopa, 1–2 g daily; guanethidine, 12.5–50.0 mg daily; prazosin hydrochloride, 1–20 mg twice a day; and phenoxybenzamine, 5–80 mg daily. The calcium channel-blocking agents are relatively new and potentially important agents in the management of Raynaud's phenomenon. Nifedipine, 10–20 mg three times daily, has shown impressive preliminary results.[110]

Therapy should be initiated at low doses and gradually adjusted upward until the desired effect is obtained or side effects supervene. The most troublesome of these side effects are orthostatic hypotension with guanethidine and methyldopa, sinus and atrial tachycardias with phenoxybenzamine, and depression and nasal stuffiness with reserpine. Less commonly, methyldopa may cause hepatic dysfunction or autoimmune hemolytic anemia. Therapy may be discontinued in warm weather to allow maximal effects when cold weather returns and to prevent undesirable cumulative side effects (e.g., tachycardias). Tolerance to these agents may develop with chronic use; however, increased dosage may overcome tolerance occasionally. Serial use of these agents rather than simultaneous mixtures is recommended, with the exception that nitroglycerin can be used locally together with another agent.

The Management of Raynaud's Syndrome

The management of Raynaud's phenomenon is aimed at increasing the patient's digital blood flow.[111] The most simple vasodilatory therapy is protection against the body's two most powerful vasoconstrictive stimuli: cold exposure and fright or frustration. The body should be protected against cold temperatures, which includes air-conditioning, as much as possible. The neck, face, and hands are well endowed with nerve endings, which, when stimulated, lead to vasoconstriction. Also, the central body should be dressed warmly (body suits) to induce a gentle and persistent state of vasodilatation. In extreme cold, battery-operated warming devices may be of benefit; it is usually not necessary to incur this degree of expense. Cessation of cigarette smoking is imperative for patients with Raynaud's phenomenon; indeed, the most difficult management problems have been with patients who, despite advice to the contrary, continued to smoke, since most therapy is ineffective in the face of continued smoking. In scleroderma patients, smoking should be managed as a life-threatening addiction.

Improvement of resting digital skin temperature and retardation of the rate of digital cooling on cold exposure have been noted after biofeedback training. Long-term maintenance of the responses, however, is variable. It is difficult to predict which vasodilator will be effective in each patient at a dose safely below the level causing side effects. Selecting the most effective agent is an extended trial-and-error process in each patient, which should be outlined to the patient at the outset and entered into with optimism and support.

Glucocorticoids

The use of glucocorticoids in the treatment of scleroderma is controversial. Despite some reports to the contrary, there is no convincing evidence that they precipitate or aggravate renal involvement. Glucocorticoids are indicated when an inflammatory process is identified (puffy skin, inflammatory myopathy, inflammatory lung disease), preferably prior to the onset of fibrosis. Prednisone (40 mg or less in divided daily dosage) for 8–12 weeks is recommended. The effect of therapy on the pathologic process should be evaluated critically following therapy. If improvement occurs, it is justifiable to continue therapy using the minimal effective dose; however, long-term corticosteroid therpay has no place in the treatment of scleroderma with the exception of active myositis. None of the vascular, visceral, or cutaneous manifestations have been shown to respond to glucocorticoids.

D-Penicillamine

Recent data indicate that in patients with rapidly progressing skin involvement, D-penicillamine may be beneficial.[112] According to experimental and clinical data, D-penicillamine inhibits intramolecular and intermolecular cross-links of collagen; this causes an increase in the amount of soluble collagen in the skin. Initial doses of 250 mg daily are suggested, with gradual increase every 2–3 months, to a maximum of 1000 mg/day. The reported incidence of side effects varies from 10 to 98 percent and includes skin rash, dyspepsia, taste disturbances, nephropathy, and bone marrow suppression. There is no evidence that penicillamine affects visceral involvement in scleroderma.

Colchicine

The use of this drug has been advocated on the basis of its ability to prevent extracellular accumulations of collagen by inhibiting the release of procollagen from fibroblasts.[113] The suggested dosage is 0.6–1.8 mg daily. This agent should be reserved for the stable patient with the chronic fibrotic stage of scleroderma. Most centers are not impressed with responses to colchicine; its safety record is, however, excellent.

Other Therapy

Recent reports on the anabolic steroid stanozolol indicate that it increases blood flow to the hands and effectively reduces the symptoms of Raynaud's phenomenon. In scleroderma, reduction of blood fibrinolytic activity has been reported, and deposits of fibrin are uniformly seen in the lumen of involved vessels. Stanozolol (5 mg twice a day orally) has been shown to stimulate the synthesis of plasminogen activator, which thereby enhances fibrinolysis.[70] Side effects (fluid retention, acne, hirsutism, and amenorrhea) can be minimized by employing cyclic courses, i.e., 3 months on therapy alternating with 2-month drug-free intervals. Plasmapheresis should be reserved for the rare patient with end-organ failure in whom all other measures have failed. Antioxidant (α-tocopherol) and immunosuppressive (azathioprine, chlorambucil, etc.) drugs have been advocated with little or no objective support for their efficacy.

MANAGEMENT OF SPECIFIC SYSTEMIC INVOLVEMENT

Trophic Ulcers and Gangrene (Peripheral Vascular System)

Digital tip infarcts are best treated with vasodilators, of which intra-arterial reserpine (0.5–1.0 mg injected directly into the radial or brachial artery) is effective. Daily intermittent cervical sympathetic blockade is also helpful in those patients whose skin temperature can be increased by this procedure. Use of topical nitroglycerin has been effective. Early aggressive local and systemic antibiotic treatment of infected ulcers is important for the prevention of chronic osteomyelitis. Surgical thoracic sympathectomy usually results in only transient relief of vasospasm and has no significant influence on the course of cutaneous or visceral sclerosis.[114] Amputation is almost never indicated due to frequent failure of healing after this procedure. Remarkably, tissue loss can regularly be minimized with prolonged conservative management.

Musculoskeletal System

Two forms of muscular involvement are seen in scleroderma. One is a slowly progressive muscular atrophy, which manifests as mild weakness and myalgia and little or no elevation in muscle enzymes (enzyme levels less than twice upper limit of normal); this form is not affected by any therapeutic approach. Less common is acute inflammatory myositis. Because it is similar to idiopathic inflammatory polymyositis in its clinical, pathologic, and electromyographic changes and corticosteroid responsiveness, prompt improvement in clinical and biochemical parameters is achieved with the use of prednisone, 1 mg/kg/day in divided doses. Steroid resistant cases may respond to azathioprine (1.5–2.0 mg/kg/day), methotrexate, or chlorambucil.

Arthralgia, arthritis, and tenosynovitis respond adequately to nonsteroidal anti-inflammatory agents.

Gastrointestinal Tract

Regular prophylactic dental care and good oral hygiene are essential, since scleroderma patients have decreased oral aperture, loosening of teeth, and xerostomia associated with Sjögren's syndrome. Symptomatic esophageal reflux is best managed by avoidance of recumbent position after meals, elevation of the head of the bed, and regular use of antacids. Cimetidine is effective in resistant cases. Prophylactic treatment is advisable and can probably prevent esophageal stricture, which, once developed, requires periodic dilatation. Metoclopramide has been shown to be effective in improving esophageal motility and increasing sphincter pressure. Malabsorption syndrome is best managed by the use of broad-spectrum antibiotics to reduce bacterial overgrowth. Cyclic intermittent courses (2 weeks/month) of tetracycline, ampicillin, and erythromycin are effective. Low-residue diet, medium-chain triglycerides, and vitamin replacement are recommended for patients with advanced intestinal atony. This approach may delay the onset of irreversible small bowel failure, which, once fully developed, is extremely difficult to manage. In a few patients, limited resection of segmental bowel involvement has proved helpful. For the majority of patients with severe gastrointestinal hypomotility, intermittent ileus, and malnutrition, home or institutionalized parenteral hyperalimentation is the only effective therapy and, in some ways, is more complicated than renal hemodialysis.

Lungs

Once pulmonary fibrosis is established radiographically, no therapy has been shown to alter its course. Theoretically, the basic approach to pharmacologic therapy is to attack the alveolitis before it causes irreversible derangement of the alveolar–capillary units, since the adult human lung cannot replenish destroyed alveolar–capillary units. The intensity of alveolitis (at the stage prior to the onset of fibrosis) correlates well with efficacy of corticosteroid treatment. Unfortunately, early detection as well as precise techniques to evaluate alveolitis in scleroderma are not available. It is important to make oxygen available to the patient once he or she demonstrates a decrease in PaO_2 with exercise to levels less than 50 mm Hg. It is critical to be aware of the development of infection, since even localized bacterial pneumonia can be fatal to such patients. In patients with pulmonary hypertension, hydralazine, isoproterenol, prazosin hydrochloride or nifedipine may be helpful. Vasodilator therapy may lead to serious adverse reactions; these include progressive renal insufficiency, symptomatic decrease in systemic arterial oxygen saturation and symptomatic hypotension, and, in some, it fails to produce consistent hemodynamic and clinical benefits.[115] Objective responses to therapy are determined most accurately by right-heart catheterization with concomitant drug administration. The reversible component of pulmonary hypertension may be small compared to the degree of fixed, irreversible vascular lesion.

Heart

Cardiac involvement in scleroderma is subtle and presents as restrictive cardiomyopathy with a high incidence of arrhythmia and AV conduction disturbances. Therapy consists of inotropic drugs, after-load reduction, and appropriate antiarrhythmic agents. Diuretics should be avoided because of their potential to produce hypovolemic renal failure.

Therapy of symptomatic acute pericarditis should be with non-steroidal anti-inflammatory drugs, such as indomethacin. In chronic cases with hemodynamic compromise, pericardiocentesis with pericardiectomy may be required. Careful observation of intravascular volume with monitoring of renal function is essential.

Kidney

Several advances have been made in the treatment of patients with malignant arterial hypertension and renal failure. In the past, this syndrome was uniformly fatal, but aggressive use of combinations of newer antihypertensive agents appears to decelerate progression of the syndrome and, in some patients, may abort the process completely. A dramatic reversal of scleroderma renal crisis by the oral angiotensin-converting enzyme inhibitor, captopril, has been reported.[116,117] This agent promotes the accumulation of bradykinin, which is normally degraded by the converting enzyme. The combined effect of captopril (inhibition of angiotensin II generation and accumulation of bradykinin) makes it the most suitable agent for this complication of scleroderma. Other agents such as hydralazine and propranolol (in doses sufficient to suppress plasma renin activity) have been effective in controlling the process. In patients with mild renal disease, it is important to maintain renal perfusion by avoiding dehydration, diuretics, hypotensive drugs, or drugs that lead to selective renal vasoconstriction. The implied role of the renin–angiotensin–aldosterone system in the pathogenesis of scleroderma renal crisis *(vide supra)* raises two interesting points. In the first place, simulation of renin should perhaps be kept to a minimum in these patients. In this connection, malignant hypertension in scleroderma has been observed in patients shortly after diuretic therapy was instituted to control blood pressure. Such volume-depleting treatment not only augments azotemia, and increases hemoconcentration, but also induces reactive rises in renin levels with increased vasoconstriction. It follows that early treatment to control vasoconstriction while protecting effective volume and tissue flow may prevent vascular damage and the renal crisis. Captopril, an ideal agent for this purpose, may be used in scleroderma as soon as there is any evidence of hypertension to protect against an insidiously increasing renin-induced vasoconstriction that could lead to an abrupt, life-threatening crisis. The protease-inhibitory properties of captopril may be useful in reducing endothelial injury in scleroderma patients. If medical management fails, intervention with hemodialysis may be lifesaving. Successful management of renal scleroderma may influence the disease manifestation in other organs, as shown by improvement of cutaneous changes, Raynaud's phenomenon, and arthralgia.[118] Agents such as captopril may eventually find a place in the general management of scleroderma.

This management outline is intended to convey the concept that each stage and site of involvement in this multistage and multisystem disorder should be considered separately. Better understanding of the mechanisms involved in the vascular and fibrotic manifestation of scleroderma will be essential to the development of effective therapy for the overall disease. At present, the greatest need is to block the specific factors that injure the endothelium and to combine these approaches with existing antiplatelet agents and other modalities.

SUMMARY

Scleroderma is both a fascinating and a frustrating disorder. Skin involvement is its hallmark; the extent of visceral involvement determines its course. In each involved organ, lesions can be characterized as immune inflammatory, followed by functional and structural alteration of the vasculature and then by a fibrotic atrophic stage. The clinical as well as the histopathologic appearance of scleroderma lesions depends on the stage of the disease at which the evaluation is done. The best current hypothesis of the pathogenesis of scleroderma is that of an immune–inflammatory response to altered endothelium of the small arteries and capillaries, this leads to endothelial injury, exposure of subendothelium, activation of platelets and the coagulation system, and migration of smooth muscle cells to the intima with eventual intimal proliferation and narrowing of the lumen. Increased collagen synthesis and deposition in the involved organ is viewed as the end result of this cycle of vascular events. The exact mechanism of fibrosis is not well understood; perhaps a lymphokine-monokine combined with other growth factors are involved in activation of interstitial fibroblasts. Recent studies support a role for humoral as well as cellular immunity in the perpetuating mechanism.

An emphasis on the immune and early vascular event in scleroderma offers many new avenues of potential therapeutic intervention, such as the prevention of Raynaud's phenomenon and the blockade of the vasculotoxic effect of renin angiotensin. Many new ideas have emerged, which, for lack of an experimental model, can only be tested in the individual patient destined to develop scleroderma. Detection of the many features of scleroderma at the earliest possible stage seems to offer the best hope for meaningful therapeutic intervention. All patients with Raynaud's phenomenon who have scleroderma-pattern nailfold capillary changes and autoimmune phenomena should be viewed as suspect to develop scleroderma and managed prospectively.

REFERENCES

1. Rodnan GP, Medsger TA Jr, Buckingham RB: Progressive systemic sclerosis-CREST syndrome: Observations on natural history and late complications in 90 patients. Arthritis Rheum 18:423 (abstract), 1975
2. Tuffanelli DL, Winkelmann RK: Systemic scleroderma: A clinical study of 727 cases. Arch Dermatol 84:359–371, 1961
3. Masi AT, Medsger TA Jr, Rodnan GP, et al.: Methods and preliminary results of the scleroderma criteria cooperative study of the American Rheumatism Association. Clin Rheum Dis 5:27–48, 1979
4. Gershwin ME, Abplanalp H, Castles JJ, et al.: Characterization of a spontaneous disease of white leghorn chickens resembling progressive systemic sclerosis (scleroderma). J Exp Med 153:1640–1659, 1981
5. Green MC, Sweet HO, Bunker LE: Tight-skin, a new mutation of the mouse causing excessive growth of connective tissue and skeleton. Am J Pathol 82:493–512, 1976
6. Sharp GC: Mixed connective tissue disease and overlap syndromes, in Kelley WN, Harris ED Jr, Ruddy S, Sledge CB (eds): Textbook of Rheumatology. Philadelphia, W. B. Saunders, 1981
7. Medsger TA Jr, Masi AT: Epidemiology of progressive systemic sclerosis. Clin Rheum Dis 5:15–25, 1979
8. LeRoy EC, Maricq HR, Kahaleh MB: Undifferentiated connective tissue syndromes. Arthritis Rheum 23:341–343, 1980
9. Kallenberg CGM, Pastoor GW, Wouda AA, et al.: Antinuclear antibodies in patients with Raynaud's phenomenon: Clinical significance of anticentromere antibodies. Ann Rheum Dis 41:382–387, 1982
10. Maricq HR, LeRoy EC, D'Angelo WA, et al.: Diagnostic potential in vivo capillary microscopy in scleroderma and related disorders. Arthritis Rheum 23:183–189, 1980
11. Harper FE, Marciq HR, Turner RE, et al.: A prospective study of Raynaud phenomenon and early connective tissue disease: A five-year report. Am J Med 72:883–888, 1982
12. Rodnan GP, Fennell RH Jr: Progressive systemic sclerosis sine scleroderma. JAMA 180:665–670, 1962
13. LeRoy EC: Scleroderma (systemic sclerosis), in Kelly WN, Harris ED Jr, Ruddy S, Sledge CB (eds): Textbook of Rheumatology. Philadelphia, W. B. Saunders, 1981
14. Rodnan GP, Lipinski E, Luksick J: Skin thickness and collagen content in progressive systemic sclerosis and localized scleroderma. Arthritis Rheum 22:130–140, 1979
15. Medsger TA Jr, Steen VO, Ziegler G, et al.: The natural history of skin involvement in progressive systemic sclerosis (PSS). Arthritis Rheum 23:720–721, 1980
16. Cole GW, Handler SJ, Burnett K: The ultrasonic evaluation of skin thickness

in scleroderma. J Clin Ultrasound 9:501–503, 1981

17. Clements PJ, Furst DE, Campion DS, et al.: Muscle disease in progressive systemic sclerosis: Diagnostic and therapeutic considerations. Arthritis Rheum 21:62–71, 1978
18. Cipoletti JF, Buckingham RB, Barnes EL, et al.: Sjögren's syndrome in progressive systemic sclerosis. Ann Intern Med 87:535–541, 1977
19. Turner R, Lipshutz W, Miller W, et al.: Esophageal dysfunction in collagen disease. Am J Med Sci 265:191–199, 1973
20. D'Angelo WA, Fries JF, Masi AT, et al.: Pathologic observation in systemic sclerosis (scleroderma): A study of fifty-eight autopsy cases and fifty-eight matched controls. Am J Med 46:428–440, 1969
21. Battle WM, Snape WJ Jr, Wright S, et al.: Abnormal colonic motility in progressive systemic sclerosis. Ann Intern Med 94:749–752, 1981
22. Crystal RG, Gadek JE, Ferrans VJ, et al.: Interstitial lung disease: Current concepts of pathogenesis, staging, and therapy. Am J Med 70:542–568, 1981
23. Bjerke RD, Tashkin DP, Clements PJ, et al.: Small airways in progressive systemic sclerosis (PSS). Am J Med 66:201–209, 1979
24. Sackner MA, Akgun N, Kimbel P, et al.: The pathophysiology of scleroderma involving the heart and respiratory system. Ann Intern Med 60:611–630, 1964
25. Young RH, Mark GJ: Pulmonary vascular changes in scleroderma. Am J Med 64:998–1004, 1978
26. Salerni R, Rodnan GP, Leon DF, et al.: Pulmonary hypertension in the CREST syndrome variant of progressive systemic sclerosis (scleroderma). Ann Intern Med 86:394–399, 1977
27. McWhorter JE IV, LeRoy EC: Pericardial disease in scleroderma (systemic sclerosis). Am J Med 57:566–575, 1974
28. Gladman DD, Gordon DA, Urowitz MB, et al.: Pericardial fluid analysis in scleroderma (systemic sclerosis). Am J Med 60:1064–1068, 1976
29. Bulkley BH, Klacsmann PG, Hutchins GM: Angina pectoris, myocardial infarction and sudden cardiac death with normal coronary arteries: A clinicopathologic study of 9 patients with progressive systemic sclerosis. Am Heart J 95:563–569, 1978
30. Weiss S, Stead EA Jr, Warren JV, et al.: Scleroderma: Heart disease with consideration of certain other visceral manifestations of scleroderma. Arch Intern Med 71:749, 1943
31. Oram S, Strokes W: The heart in scleroderma. Br Heart J 23:243, 1961
32. Botstein GR, LeRoy EC: Primary heart disease in systemic sclerosis (scleroderma): Advances in clinical and pathologic features, pathogenesis, and new therapeutic approaches. Am Heart J 102:913–919, 1981
33. Roberts NK, Cabeen WR Jr, Moss J, et al.: The prevalence of conduction defects and cardiac arrhythmias in progressive systemic sclerosis. Ann Intern Med 94:38–40, 1981
34. Gottdiener JS, Moutsopoulos HM, Decker JL: Echocardiographic identification of cardiac abnormality in scleroderma and related disorders. Am J Med 66:391–398, 1979
35. Kahaleh MB, LeRoy EC: Progressive systemic sclerosis: Kidney involvement. Clin Rheum Dis 5:167–184, 1979
36. Gavras H, Gavras I, Cannon PJ, et al.: Is elevated plasma renin activity of prognostic importance in progressive systemic sclerosis? Arch Intern Med 137:1554–1558, 1977
37. Gordon MB, Klein I, Dekker A, et al.: Thyroid disease in progressive systemic sclerosis: Increased frequency of glandular fibrosis and hypothyroidism. Ann Intern Med 95:431–435, 1981
38. Sheldon WB, Lurie DP, Maricq HR, et al.: Three siblings with scleroderma (systemic sclerosis) and two with Raynaud's phenomenon from a single kindred. Arthritis Rheum 24:668–676, 1981
39. Clements PJ, Opelz G, Terasaki PI, et al.: Associations of HLA antigen A9 with progressive systemic sclerosis (scleroderma). Tissue Antigens 11:357–361, 1978
40. Rabin BS, Rodnan GP, Bassion S, et al.: HLA antigens in progressive sys-

temic sclerosis (scleroderma). Arthritis Rheum 18:381–382, 1975

41. Lynch CJ, Singh G, Whiteside TL, et al.: Histocompatibility antigens in progressive systemic sclerosis (PSS; Scleroderma). J Clin Immunol 2:314–318, 1982
42. Pan SF, Rodnan GP, Deutsch M, et al.: Chromosomal abnormalities in progressive systemic sclerosis (scleroderma) with consideration of radiation effects. J Lab Clin Med 86:300–308, 1975
43. Emerit I: Chromosomal abnormalities in progressive systemic sclerosis. Clin Rheum Dis 5:201–214, 1979
44. Norton WL, Nardo JM: Vascular disease in progressive systemic sclerosis (scleroderma). Ann Intern Med 73:317–324, 1970
45. Fleischmajer R, Perlish JS: Capillary alterations in scleroderma. J Am Acad Dermatol 2:161–170, 1980
46. Fleischmajer R, Perlish JS: [^{3}H]Thymidine labeling of dermal endothelial cells in scleroderma. J Invest Dermatol 69:379–382, 1977
47. Kahaleh MB, Sherer GK, LeRoy EC: Endothelial injury in scleroderma. J Exp Med 149:1326–1335, 1979
48. Kahaleh MB, LeRoy EC: Endothelial injury in scleroderma: A protease mechanism. J Lab Clin Med 101:553–560, 1983
49. Ross R, Glomset J, Kariya B, et al.: A platelet-dependent serum factor that stimulates the proliferation of arterial smooth muscle cells in vitro. Proc Natl Acad Sci USA 71:1207–1210, 1974
50. Wechezak AR, Mansfield PB, Way SA: Platelet interaction with cultured endothelial cells following in vitro injury. Artery 1:507–517, 1975
51. Green D: Role of the von Willebrand factor in atherogenesis. Artery 5:262–272, 1979
52. Kahaleh MB, Osborn I, LeRoy EC: Increased factor VIII/von Willebrand factor antigen and von Willebrand factor activity in scleroderma and in Raynaud's phenomenon. Ann Intern Med 94:482–484, 1981
53. Brinkhous KM, Sultzer DL, Reddick RL, et al.: Elevated plasma von Willebrand factor (vWf) levels as an index of acute endothelial injury: Use of a hypotonic injury model in rats. Fed Proc 39:630, 1980
54. Fuster V, Bowie EJW, Lewis JC, et al.: Resistance to arteriosclerosis in pigs with von Willebrand's disease: Spontaneous and high cholesterol diet-induced arteriosclerosis. J Clin Invest 61:722–730, 1978
55. Harker LA, Ross R, Glomset JA: The role of endothelial cell injury and platelet response in atherogenesis. Thromb Haemostas 39:312–321, 1978
56. Kahaleh MB, Osborn I, LeRoy EC: Elevated levels of circulating platelet aggregates and beta-thromboglobulin in scleroderma. Ann Intern Med 96:610–613, 1982
57. Niewiarowski S: Proteins secreted by the platelet. Thromb Haemostas 38:924–938, 1977
58. Doyle DJ, Chesterman CN, Cade JF, et al.: Plasma concentrations of platelet-specific proteins correlated with platelet survival. Blood 55:82–84, 1980
59. Hope W, Martin TJ, Chesterman CN, et al.: Human B-thromboglobulin inhibits PGI_2 production and binds to a specific site in bovine aortic endothelial cells. Nature 282:210–212, 1979
60. Case records of the Massachusetts General Hospital: Weekly clinicopathological exercises. Case 34–1978. N Engl J Med 299:466–474, 1978
61. Sakariassen KS, Bolhuis PA, Sixma JJ: Platelet adherence to subendothelium of human arteries in pulsatile and steady flow. Thromb Res 19:547–559, 1980
62. Gratwick GM, Klein R, Sergent JS, et al.: Fibrinogen turnover in progressive systemic sclerosis. Arthritis Rheum 21:343–347, 1978
63. Furey NL, Schmid FR, Kwaan HC, et al.: Arterial thrombosis in scleroderma. Br J Dermatol 93:683–693, 1975
64. Holland CD, Jayson MIV: Venous blood fibrinolysis and fibrinolytic potential in Raynaud's phenomenon (RP) and systemic sclerosis (SS). Ann Rheum Dis 40:518–519, 1981
65. Cherry GW, Ryan TJ, Ellis JE: Decreased fibrinolysis in reperfused ischaemic tissue. Thromb Diath Haemorrh 32:659–664, 1974

66. Kadish JL: Fibrin and atherogenesis: A hypothesis. Atherosclerosis 33:409–413, 1979
67. LeRoy EC, Downey JA, Cannon PJ: Skin capillary blood flow in scleroderma. J Clin Invest 50:930–939, 1971
68. Martin MFR, Dowd PM, Ring EFJ, et al.: Prostaglandin E_1 infusions for vascular insufficiency in progressive systemic sclerosis. Ann Rheum Dis 40:350–354, 1981
69. Hossman V, Heinen A, Auel H, et al.: A randomized, placebo controlled trial of prostacyclin (PGI_2) in peripheral arterial disease. Thromb Res 22:481–490, 1981
70. Jarrett PEM, Morland M, Browse NL: Treatment of Raynaud's phenomenon by fibrinolytic enhancement. Br Med J 2:523–525, 1978
71. LeRoy EC: The connective tissue in scleroderma. Coll Rel Res 1:301–308, 1981
72. Fleischmajer R, Gay S, Perlish JS, et al.: Immunoelectron microscopy of type III collagen in normal and scleroderma skin. J Invest Dermatol 75:189–191, 1980
73. Gay RE, Buckingham RB, Prince RK, et al.: Collagen types synthesized in dermal fibroblast cultures from patients with early progressive systemic sclerosis. Arthritis Rheum 23:190–196, 1980
74. Lovell CR, Nicholls AC, Duance VC, et al.: Characterization of dermal collagen in systemic sclerosis. Br J Dermatol 100:359–369, 1979
75. LeRoy EC: Increased collagen synthesis by scleroderma skin fibroblasts in vitro: A possible defect in the regulation or activation of the scleroderma fibroblast. J Clin Invest 54:880–889, 1974
76. Kuhn K, Wiestner M, Krieg T, et al.: Structure and function of the amino terminal propeptide of type I and III collagen. Connect Tissue Res 10:43–50, 1982
77. Fleischmajer R, Dessau W, Timpl R, et al.: Immunofluorescence analysis of collagen, fibronectin, and basement membrane protein in scleroderma skin. J Invest Dermatol 75:270–274, 1980
78. Botstein GR, Sherer GK, LeRoy EC: Fibroblast selection in scleroderma: An alternate model of fibrosis. Arthritis Rheum 25:189–195, 1982
79. LeRoy EC, Kahaleh MB, Mercurio S: A fibroblast mitogen present in scleroderma but not control sera: Inhibition by proteinase inhibitors. Rheumatol Int 3:35–38, 1983
80. Brady AH: Collagenase in scleroderma. J Clin Invest 56:1175–1180, 1975
81. Uitto J, Bauer EA, Eisen AZ: Scleroderma: Increased biosynthesis of triple-helical type I and type III procollagens associated with unaltered expression of collagenase by skin fibroblasts in culture. J Clin Invest 64:921–930, 1979
82. Krane S: Collagen degradation. Connect Tissue Res 10:51–59, 1982
83. Husson JM, Le Go A, Engler R, et al.: Immunochemical study on serum proteins in systemic sclerosis. Biomedicine 26:182–187, 1977
84. Tan EM, Rodnan GP, Garcia I, et al.: Diversity of antinuclear antibodies in progressive systemic sclerosis. Arthritis Rheum 23:617–625, 1980
85. Farber SJ, Bole GG: Antibodies to components of extractable nuclear antigen. Arch Intern Med 136:425–431, 1976
86. Alarcon-Segovia D, Fishbein E: Immunochemical characterization of the anti-RNA antibodies found in scleroderma and systemic lupus erythematosus: I. Differences in reactivity in poly (U) and poly (A)-poly (U). J Immunol 115:28–31, 1975
87. Fritzler MJ, Kinsella TD, Garbutt E: The CREST syndrome: A distinct serologic entity with anticentromere antibodies. Am J Med 69:520–526, 1980
88. Brentnall TJ, Kenneally D, Barnett AJ, et al.: Autoantibodies to fibroblasts in scleroderma. J Clin Lab Immunol 8:9–12, 1982
89. Mackel AM, DeLustro F, Harper FE, et al.: Antibodies to collagen in scleroderma. Arthritis Rheum 25:522–531, 1982
90. Fleischmajer R, Perlish JS, West WP: Ultrastructure of cutaneous cellular infiltrates in scleroderma. Arch Dermatol 113:1661–1666, 1977
91. Alarcon-Segovia D, Palacios R, De Kasep GI: Human postthymic precursor cells in health and disease: VIII. Immunoregulatory circuits of the peripheral blood mononuclear cells from

patients with progressive systemic sclerosis. J Clin Lab Immunol 5:143–148, 1981
92. Hughes P, Holt S, Rowell NR, et al.: The relationship of defective cell-mediated immunity to visceral disease in systemic sclerosis. Clin Exp Immunol 28:233–240, 1977
93. Wright JK, Hughes P, Rowell NR, et al.: Antibody-dependent and phytohaemagglutinin-induced lymphocyte cytotoxicity in systemic sclerosis. Clin Exp Immunol 36:175–182, 1979
94. Keystone EC, Lau C, Gladman DD, et al.: Immunoregulatory T-cell subpopulations in patients with scleroderma using monoclonal antibodies. Clin Exp Immunol 48:443–488, 1982
95. Currie S, Saunders M, Knowles M: Immunological aspects of systemic sclerosis: In vitro activity of lymphocytes from patients with the disorder. Br J Dermatol 84:400, 1970
96. Kondo H, Rabin BS, Rodnan GP: Cutaneous antigen-stimulating lymphokine production by lymphocytes of patients with progressive systemic sclerosis (scleroderma). J Clin Invest 58:1388–1394, 1976
97. Kondon H, Rabin BS, Rodnan GP: Stimulation of lymphocyte reactivity by a low molecular weight cutaneous antigen in patients with progressive systemic sclerosis (scleroderma). J Rheumatol 6:30–37, 1979
98. Shulman HM, Sullivan KM, Weiden PL, et al.: Chronic graft-versus-host syndrome in man: A long-term clinicopathologic study of 20 Seattle patients. Am J Med 69:204–217, 1980
99. Kumagai Y, Abe C, Shiokawa Y: Scleroderma after cosmetic surgery: Four cases of human adjuvant disease. Arthritis Rheum 22:532–537, 1979
100. Kahaleh MB, DeLustro F, Osborn I, et al.: Scleroderma mononuclear cells inhibit endothelial cells and stimulate fibroblasts through soluble mediator(s). Clin Res 29:166A, 1981
101. DeLustro F, LeRoy EC: Characterization of the release of human monocyte regulators of fibroblast proliferation. J Reticuloendothel Soc 31:295–305, 1982
102. Bitterman PB, Rennard SI, Hunninghake GW, et al.: Human alveolar macrophage growth factor for fibroblasts: Regulation and partial characterization. J Clin Invest 70:806–822, 1982
103. Shulman LE: Diffuse fasciitis with eosinophilia: A new syndrome. Trans Assoc Am Physicians 88:70–86, 1975
104. Jablonska S: Scleroderma and Pseudoscleroderma. Warsaw: Polish Medical Pub, 1975
105. Selikoff IJ, Hammond EC (eds): Toxicity of vinyl chloride-polyvinyl chloride. Ann NY Acad Sci 246:1–337, 1975
106. Finch WR, Rodnan GP, Buckingham RB, et al.: Bleomycin-induced scleroderma. J Rheumatol 7:651–659, 1980
107. Palestine RF, Millns JL, Spigel GT, et al.: Skin manifestations of pentazocine abuse. J Am Acad Dermatol 2:47–55, 1980
108. Fleischmajer R, Pollock JL: Progressive systemic sclerosis: Pseudoscleroderma. Clin Rheum Dis 5:243–261, 1979
109. Fries JF, Lindgren JA, Bull JM: Scleroderma-like lesions and the carcinoid syndrome. Arch Intern Med 131:550–553, 1973
110. Smith CD, McKendry RJ: Controlled trial of nifedipine in the treatment of Raynaud's phenomenon. Lancet Dec 11, 1299–1301, 1982
111. Harper FE, LeRoy EC: Raynaud's phenomenon and scleroderma. Compr Ther 7:45–51, 1981
112. Steen VD, Medsger TA Jr, Rodnan GP: D-penicillamine therapy in progressive systemic sclerosis (scleroderma): A retrospective analysis. Ann Intern Med 97:652–659, 1982
113. Alarcon-Segovia D, Ibanez G, Kershenobich D, et al.: Treatment of scleroderma by modification of collagen metabolism: A double-blind trial with colchicine—placebo. J Rheumatol Suppl 1:97, 1974
114. Chamberlain J, Macpherson AIS: Cervico-dorsal sympathectomy for Raynaud's syndrome. JR Coll Surg Edinb 19:228–232, 1974
115. Packer M, Greenberg B, Massie B, et al.: Deleterious effects of hydralazine in patients with pulmonary hypertension. N Engl J Med 306:1326–1331, 1982

116. Lopez-Ovejero JA, Saal SD, D'Angelo WA, et al.: Medical intelligence: Reversal of vascular and renal crises of scleroderma by oral angiotensis-converting-enzyme blockade. N Engl J Med 300:1417–1419, 1977
117. Whitman HH III, Case DB, Laragh JH, et al.: Variable response to oral angiotensin-converting-enzyme blockade in hypertensive scleroderma patients. Arthritis Rheum 25:241–248, 1982
118. Barker DJ, Farr MJ: Resolution of cutaneous manifestations of systemic sclerosis after haemodialysis: Case report and discussion. Br Med J 1:501, 1976

James R. Klinenberg
Ronald Reichman
Phillip J. Clements

4

Investigational Therapy for Rheumatoid Arthritis

CYTOTOXIC THERAPY

The era of experimentation with cytotoxic therapy for rheumatoid arthritis (RA) began in 1950 following a report by Diaz, which described improvement in 14 patients with RA who were treated with nitrogen mustard. During the years that have followed, four agents have been studied almost exclusively for use in the treatment of RA: azathioprine (AZA) and its metabolite, 6-mercaptopurine (6-MP); chlorambucil (CHLOR), cyclophosphamide (CPA); and methotextrate (MTX). Although 6-MP was studied extensively in the earlier years, its clinical use has markedly declined and has been supplanted by AZA, which is less toxic.

These cytotoxic drugs have many properties, but the property of "immunosuppression" has captured the imagination of many investigators. It is appropriate, therefore, to review briefly what is known about cytotoxic-induced immunosuppression in man and how it may relate to the treatment of RA (Table 4-1).[1-21] Since CHLOR has not been studied in this regard, the following discussion will focus primarily on AZA, 6-MP, CPA, and MTX.

Immunosuppression by Cytotoxic Drugs

Simplistically, the immune response can be divided into humoral and cell-mediated responses and both can be subdivided into primary and secondary phases. Primary responses are initiated by "new" antigenic stimuli

PROGRESS IN CLINICAL RHEUMATOLOGY VOL. I ISBN 0-8089-1646-7

Table 4-1
Summary of Immunosuppressive Effects of Cytotoxic Agents as Determined in Humans

Immune function studied	Drug effect in man	Antigenic stimulus or method of assessing response	References
Humoral			
Primary response (IgM)	CPA, AZA (6-MP), MTX may prevent, prolong, or delay response. MTX may enhance	Vi antigen, tularemia, pneumococcus, flagellin, KLH, plague, tetanus	1–9
Switchover from IgM to IgG	CPA, AZA (6-MP), MTX may prevent or blunt	Vi antigen, KLH, flagellin	2,4,7,8
Secondary or anamnestic response (IgG)	Although CPA, AZA (6-MP), MTX may decrease, they usually exert little suppression	Diphtheria, pneumococcus, mumps, measles, Candida, influenza A & B, tetanus	7,8,10–13
Cell-medicated (CMI)			
Primary induction	CPA, AZA (6-MP), MTX may prevent	Tularemia, KLH, DNCB	1,2,5–7

Recall of established CMI	All usually exert little suppression although CPA and CHLOR may suppress skin tests	Standard battery of skin tests (PPD, mumps, Candida, trichophyton, coccidioidin)	1,5,6,8,9,11,14–16
Proliferative response (in vitro)	CPA, CHLOR, MTX often suppress but AZA (6-MP) usually exerts little effect	Thymidine uptake in response to PHA, PWM, specific antigens	5,10,11,14,15,17,18
Induction of tolerance	CPA and AZA (6-MP) can induce. No effect shown by MTX or CHLOR in man.	Vi antigen, plague, allogeneic bone marrow or kidney	1,18
Prolongation of graft survival	CPA and AZA (6-MP) can prolong MTX and CHLOR not demonstrated effective in man	Allogeneic bone marrow or kidney	1,19,20
Anti-inflammatory	CPA, AZA (6-MP) MTX have anti-inflammatory properties	Rebuck skin window	21

while secondary responses follow reexposure or rechallenge with booster doses of antigen. Antibody formed in response to a new antigenic stimulus is usually and predominantly of the IgM class; it usually reaches peak levels within several weeks. During the first few weeks, some IgG antibody is formed, but it initially is in small quantities. Shortly after the IgM antibody levels peak and begin to fall, the levels of IgG antibody begin to rise, and eventually IgG becomes the predominant class ("switchover" from IgM to IgG). If the same antigen is readministered at a later time, the antibody response that results is predominantly of the IgG class (secondary response). In the secondary or anamnestic response, the levels of antibody usually reach a higher peak and rise more rapidly than did the antibody in the primary response. New antigens may also "induce" cell-mediated immunity (CMI), while rechallenge with the same antigen at a later time will evoke a recall of established CMI (delayed hypersensitivity). As a group, the cytotoxics are more likely to modify or abrogate a primary immune response (both humoral and CMI) than a secondary response, which is usually resistant to modification by these drugs. In addition, they may prevent or delay the normal switchover of antibody response from IgM to IgG.

With the possible exception of AZA (6-MP), the cytotoxics may suppress the in vitro proliferative response to specific mitogen or specific antigenic stimulation (considered by some to be a measure of CMI).

Transplantation of an allogeneic organ (i.e., bone marrow, skin, kidney) will normally result in an immune response (both humoral and CMI), which is directed at rejection of the organ. Of the cytotoxics, only AZA (6-MP) and CPA have proven to be clinically useful in prolonging graft survival, partly through the induction of tolerance (a state in which the recipient, on repeated exposure to the foreign organ or antigen, mounts no immune response) or through suppression of the resulting immune or inflammatory response. The cytotoxics are most effective when given just prior to or at the time of organ transplantation. Once the immune response has become established, however, it is much more difficult to induce tolerance or to suppress the immune response.

The cytotoxics have also been shown to have anti-inflammatory properties and this may suppress the inflammatory response that often accompanies CMI (again CHLOR has not been well studied), as in the tuberculin reaction. The suppression of the inflammatory response thus has undoubtedly been misconstrued at times as suppression of CMI rather than simply an anti-inflammatory response.

The degree of immunosuppression produced by the cytotoxic drugs has been extremely variable and quite dependent on a number of factors, some of which are listed next (with illustrated examples):

1. *The drug*. Induction of tolerance and prolongation of graft survival has been clearly demonstrated for AZA (6-MP) and CPA but not for CHLOR

or MTX. Suppression of established skin test reactivity is rarely seen with AZA (6-MP) or MTX but can be seen with CPA and CHLOR.

2. *Dose and route of administration of drug.* Increasing the dose of drug usually results in greater degrees of immunosuppression.
3. *Duration of drug therapy.* Virtually no suppression of the primary humoral or CMI (skin test reactivity) response to Keyhole-limpet hemocyanin (KLH) was seen in subjects treated for 2 weeks with CPA at a dose of 1.0 mg/kg/day, whereas 7 of the 9 subjects treated with CPA for many months at a dose of 50–125 mg/day failed to develop humoral or skin test reactivity to KLH.
4. *The nature of the antigenic stimulus.* As mentioned above, the immune response to a new antigen is more easily suppressed than the response to a booster stimulus.
5. *Timing of antigen administration in relation to drug administration.* In general, the cytotoxics most effectively suppress the immune response when antigen is administered 1–2 days prior to beginning cytotoxic therapy. CPA is the only one of the four which may also be somewhat effective in suppressing the primary immune response when it is begun 1–2 days after the administration of antigen.
6. *State of health of the subject.* Many diseases themselves may modify the subject's ability to respond immunologically. For example, systemic lupus erythematosus (SLE) patients treated with AZA and steroids have a response to pneumococcal antigens that is less than normal, but the response is equivalent to that seen in SLE patients not receiving AZA. Established skin reactivity to common antigens is reduced in many subjects with acute leukemia and is often improved following a cytotoxic-induced remission. Renal-transplant recipients treated with AZA and prednisone did not develop an IgG response to flagellin, whereas most patients with autoimmune disease treated with AZA and prednisone developed both an IgM and an IgG response to flagellin.
7. *Concomitant use of other drugs.* The concomitant use of more than one cytotoxic agent in cancer chemotherapy is often more immunosuppressive than any one of the agents alone.

Since RA is associated with immunologic abnormalities of long duration (some of which may be of pathogenetic importance), it has seemed reasonable to treat the disease with drugs that have immunosuppressive properties. The drugs reviewed here, however, have been shown to be most effective in preventing or suppressing a primary immune response and in inducing tolerance to a new antigen. They have not been particularly effective in suppressing a preexisting immune response or inducing a tolerance to antigens. It would seem, thus, that although the cytotoxics do have immunosuppressive properties (properties that must be recognized when the drugs are used clinically), the property of immunosuppression offers an incomplete explanation for the efficacy of these drugs in the treatment of RA.

Probably more pertinent to the discussion of the mechanism of action of the cytotoxics is that their major effects are exerted through their capacity to interfere in many of the biosynthetic reactions necessary for the growth and replication of cells.[22–24] AZA and 6-MP are purine analogs that prevent interconversion of purine bases by suppressing synthesis of adenine and guanine and that inhibit the first step of de novo synthesis of purine bases. The alkylating agents CHLOR and CPA cross-link DNA and proteins, which thus prevents cell replication. MTX inhibits dihydrofolate reductase, which prevents the synthesis of two precursors essential to the formation of DNA (thymidylic acid and inosinic acid). Although each of the cytotoxics thus acts in slightly different ways, they all act to inhibit cell division. Inhibition of cell division then results in eventual death of the remaining cells, which explains the derivation of the term "cytotoxic." This mechanism of action also suggests that cell death and the interruption of important metabolic pathways are important aspects of the actions of the drugs.

CLINICAL STUDIES

AZA and CPA have undergone extensive studies in the treatment of RA. In Table 4-2[22,25,26] are summarized the important controlled and uncontrolled studies, which have examined the use of CPA and AZA in RA. There are, in addition, several recent reviews that discuss and interpret these studies and provide guidelines for their clinical use in RA.[22,24,25] Both drugs have been found to provide significant clinical improvement in the activity of the arthritis, to retard bone destruction, to ameliorate some of the nonarticular complications such as interstitial lung disease and cutaneous ulcers, and to reduce the need for concomitant corticosteroids. Patients who have shown initial improvement often continue to maintain this improvement for several years with continued use of the drugs. Once the drugs are discontinued, however, the disease process often reactivates within the next year. AZA has already been approved by the Food and Drug Administration (FDA) for use in RA and is really no longer an experimental medication. CPA, on the other hand, has been shown to be efficacious in RA, but its toxicity will undoubtedly keep its use relegated to the experimental treatment of those subjects with severe refractory disease.

CHLOR has received little attention in the United States for treatment of RA. Its published use has been limited primarily to France and Australia. Although numerous uncontrolled studies of CHLOR have been reported, only one controlled study has appeared. Its use in RA has recently been reviewed by Amor and Meoy.[23] Characteristically, CHLOR has been given in initial doses of 0.2 mg/kg/day until the arthritis responds or until leukopenia has appeared. At that point, the drug has either been discontinued or it has been continued in doses necessary to maintain the white blood cell count

Table 4-2
Summary of Controlled Trials and of Long-Term Studies of Cytotoxic Agents in Rheumatoid Arthritis

Drug	Dose (mg/kg/d)	Months on drug	Comments	Reporting investigator* (Year reported)
AZA versus placebo				
AZA (25)†	2.5	12	AZA was steroid sparing as compared to PLACEBO	Mason 1969
PLAC (24)	—			
AZA (18)	3.0	6	AZA was more effective than PLACEBO	Levy 1972
PLAC (18)	—			
AZA (17)	2.5	4	AZA was more effective than PLACEBO	Urowitz 1973
PLAC (17)	—			
AZA (30)	1.5–2.0	3	AZA was more effective than PLACEBO	Goebel 1976
PLAC (30)	—			
CPA versus placebo				
CPA (20)	2.0	8	CPA at 2.0 mg/kg/d more effective than placebo clinically and in retarding bone destruction radiographically.	Cooperating Clinics 1970
PLAC (20)	—‡			
CPA (11)	1.8	11	CPA more effective than PLACEBO	Townes 1976
PLAC (11)	—			

(continued)

Table 4-2 (continued)

Drug	Dose (mg/kg/d)	Months on drug	Comments	Reporting investigator* (Year reported)
Dose responses of CPA and of AZA				
AZA (24)	2.0–2.5	6	Both doses of AZA equally effective	Urowitz 1974
AZA	1.0–1.25			
CPA (10)	0.7–1.0	12	Effect of CPA at this dose was no better than PLACEBO	Lidsky 1973
PLAC (11)	—			
CPA (38)	1.78	8	Lower dose CPA as effective as the higher dose CPA	Williams 1980
CPA (37)	0.75			
Comparisons among cytotoxic drugs and/or other antirheumatic drugs				
CPA (18)	1.5–2.0	6	AZA and CPA equally effective and significantly better than placebo	Levy 1975
AZA (24)	3.0			
PLAC (42)	—			
CPA (13)	1.1	6	CPA in low dose (1.1 mg/kg/d) + prednisone significantly better than prednisone + placebo	Smyth 1975
PLAC (16)	—			
CPA (39)	1.5	18	All equally effective clinically. AZA and CPA more effective than gold in retarding bone destruction.	Currey 1974
AZA (44)	2.5			
Gold (38)	50mg q month			
AZA (33)	2.5	12	Both equally efficacious and with equal frequency of toxicity	Berry 1976
D-penicillin (32)	1gm/d			

AZA (11) Gold (11) Chloroquine (11)	1.8 50mg/q week 250mg/d	6	All equally effective with equal low frequency of toxicity	Dwosh 1977
Long-term studies with cytotoxic drugs in RA (controlled and uncontrolled studies)				
AZA (27)	2.5	30	Steroid sparing by AZA was mantained	Harris 1971
AZA (12)	1.5–2.5	40	Eleven of twelve maintained improvement	Hunter 1975
AZA (16)	1.0–2.5	36	15 of 16 deteriorated when AZA blindly withdrawn	Cade 1976
AZA (21)	1.4	30	Initial improvement in 12 subjects, of whom 10 maintained this improvement for 30 months	Pinals 1976
CPA (108)	—	6–72	95 had partial or complete remissions	Fosdick 1969
CPA (32)	108mg/d	19	Of 32 patients who improved during 19 months of CPA, 16 maintained remission for 41 months following withdrawal of CPA	Stojanovic 1978

*Each study is reviewed and fully referenced in one of the following articles (Davis et al[25]; Styanovic et al[26]; Bunch and O'Duffy[22].
†( ) = number of subjects receiving drug
‡Placebo consisted of CPA at 0.2 mg/kg/d

between 2000 and 4000/cm³ (with the usual dosage ranging between 2.5 mg 3 times a week and 5 mg/day). Reports suggest that between 50 and 75 percent of RA patients so treated have at least a partial response and that it may take a minimum of 4–6 months to see a significant response. Subjects who respond favorably and who can tolerate the medication often have a continuing good response as long as the medication is administered. Once the medication is discontinued, however, the disease may reactivate but the chlorambucil-induced response often is maintained for a longer period than the responses that follow withdrawal of AZA or CPA.

MTX has recently received a lot of attention as an experimental treatment of RA but no controlled studies have yet appeared.[27,28] Several investigators have reported that about two-thirds of the patients have had a favorable clinical response within the first 6–12 weeks at a dose of 7.5–15.0 mg MTX given once weekly in 3 divided doses 12 hours apart. Although the investigators have evaluated liver enzyme determinations as an index of hepatic toxicity, many have not assiduously used liver biopsy to look for the most feared adverse effect of MTX, namely, hepatic fibrosis and cirrhosis. This is in spite of the fact that the dermatologic literature has recently documented that MTX given in these low doses once weekly has induced hepatic cirrhosis and fibrosis, usually after the cumulative dose has exceeded 1.5 g (Table 4-3).[29–33] The dermatologic studies cited previously also have clearly shown that liver enzyme levels have not correlated with hepatic fibrosis or cirrhosis and will not, therefore, substitute for liver biopsy. In contradistinction to what occurs following discontinuance of the other three cytotoxics, the activity of the arthritis often returns fairly quickly to predrug levels when MTX is discontinued.

TOXICITY

The major reluctance to the widespread use of the cytotoxics in RA has been their toxicity, both evidenced and potential.[22–24,28] All four drugs can cause bone marrow dysfunction, nausea and other gastrointestinal (GI) distress, and, occasionally, rashes. Liver toxicity is seen primarily with MTX and AZA. AZA causes temporary cholestatic liver dysfunction, while MTX produces permanent hepatic fibrosis and cirrhosis. There is overwhelming evidence that the use of the alkalating agents CPA and CHLOR in the treatment of rheumatic diseases results in neoplasia, particularly of the hematologic system and the skin, while there is no evidence that MTX results in malignancy. Whether AZA use in the rheumatic diseases is associated with malignancy is controversial. The fact that the use of AZA in transplantation therapy is definitely associated with a considerable increase in malignancy is worrisome and should keep all its prescribers alert to the possibility that malignancy may occur in subjects receiving AZA. The alkylating agents

Table 4-3
Studies in Which Patients (Most Having Psoriasis) Underwent one or more Liver Biopsies Before (pre-MTX) and/or During (post-MTX) Low-Dose Intermittent Methotrexate Therapy

Reference	No. of patients	Dosage schedule	Route of administration	Mean cumulative dose (mg)	Mean treatment period (mos)	Average monthly dose (mg)	No. with fibrosis		No. with cirrhosis	
							Pre-MTX	Post-MTX	Pre-MTX	Post-MTX
30	56	Single-dose: 10–50 mg/wk; or divided-dose: 7.5–22.5 mg/wk*	IM, PO	963	15	64	—	—	1	4
31	28	Single-dose: 5–25 mg/wk	PO	(227–6698)†	(8–84)†	—	—	↑ in 4	—	No ↑
32	15	Divided-dose: 7.5–22.5 mg/wk*	PO	—	<24	—	0	6	0	0
32	19	Single-dose: ≤25 mg/wk	PO	—	<24	—	0	3	0	0
33	88	Single-dose: ≤25 mg/wk	PO	1733	26	67	0	6	0	5
34	25	Single-dose: ≤25 mg/wk	PO	1760	30	59	2	3	0	0

— = Data not available in reference
* = Divided dose was administered as 2.5–7.5 mg q12 hours × 3 doses once a week
† = Range of values shown since mean values were not given in reference

frequently produce sterility (which is often permanent), whereas AZA and MTX do not. MTX is the only one of the four drugs that is definitely teratogenetic, and pregnancy is absolutely contraindicated during MTX therapy. The evidence that CPA and CHLOR may be teratogenic is minimal, but patients should nevertheless avoid pregnancy while taking any of these drugs. AZA seems to be free of obvious teratogenicity. All four agents have been suspected of producing chronic interstitial pulmonary disease in low incidence. MTX may cause an acute pulmonary toxicity with cough, dyspnea, pulmonary infiltrates, and systemic symptoms. Although this acute complication is usually transitory and remits with minimal residue, it can be serious and result in fatality.

COMBINATION THERAPY

The presently reviewed cytotoxic agents have not been the panacea initially promised, possibly because they have failed to provide the efficacy necessary to justify the significant toxicity associated with their use. A small amount of experimentation has been performed by use of other cytotoxic agents such as nitrogen mustard and cytosine arabinoside, but these, too, have failed to justify their toxicity.

For that reason, the search continues for more efficacious therapy. Recently there has been some interest in the concomitant use of two or more disease-modifying antirheumatic drugs (DMARDs). For example, Bunch and Duffy[22] recently reported that the concomitant use of penicillamine and hydroxychloroquine failed to provide efficacy as good as either drug alone. The Cooperating Clinics for the Systematic Study of the Rheumatic Diseases is optimistically considering a protocol that would evaluate the concomitant use of AZA and gold. Their study to the contrary,[22] it is hoped that two or more DMARDs used concomitantly early in the disease will halt the progression of RA in a manner superior to the effects of single agents alone.

PHYSICAL AGENT MODALITIES

Experimental treatment of intractable, progressive RA has been attempted with several modalities, which include the use of physical agent modalities to reduce lymphocyte and, particularly, thymus-dependent lymphocyte populations. These include thoracic duct drainage (TDD), apheresis (this includes plasmapheresis (PP), lymphopheresis, lymphoplasmapheresis (LPP), and, most recently, cryopheresis, which is not really a physical method for treating T-lymph populations), and total lymphoid irradiation.

Thoracic Duct Drainage

Although "bloodletting" has been advocated as a therapeutic modality for centuries, its rationale for use has been rejected by modern medicine as barbaric and adversely affecting patients. Despite this widely held belief, more subtle forms of bloodletting have played an active role in the therapy of numerous diseases in the past decades, most obviously seen in renal failure (hemodialysis) and various drug overdoses (exchange transfusions).

A strong suspicion that lymphocytes played an important role in the immune system led to various attempts at selectively removing lymphocytes from man and animal. One of these methods used has been to cannulate the thoracic duct, which is responsible for returning lymphocytes from tissue to the circulation (Fig. 4-1). Early experiments demonstrated increased survival time of skin grafts in rats and of kidney transplantation in both dogs and man.

In 1964, Dumont et al.[34] diverted the return circulation of lymph in rats and placed homologous skin grafts under the renal capsule. A marked prolongation of graft survival time was noted but only if the lymph was diverted to the GI tract and thus excreted, as opposed to being returned to the circulation. In other rats, the thoracic duct was ligated, without diversion of the lymph flow; in these animals, no increase in graft survival was noted compared to controls. Dumont et al.[34] noted, without further discussion, that

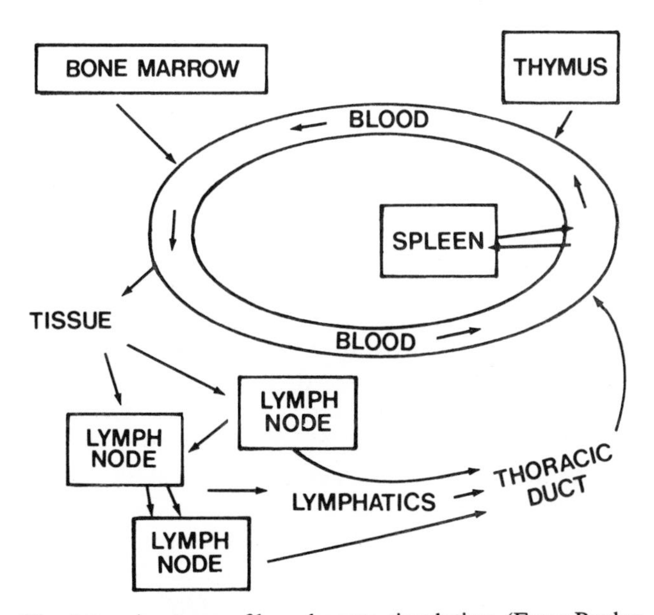

Fig. 4-1. Anatomy of lymphocyte circulation. (From Paulus HE: Prolonged thoracic-duct drainage in rheumatoid arthritis and systemic lupus erythematosus. West J Med 4:309–324, 1979. With permission.)

although the abdominal lymph cannulation became occluded within 9 days, the skin homografts survived for as long as 3½ months. This would suggest that external diversion of lymphatic return may produce lengthy immunosuppression or, alternatively, that "protection" from cells or other constituents of lymph during the crucial, first exposure to foreign antigens may induce lasting immunoacceptance of these antigens.

Dumont et al. also reported in the same paper on the diagnostic and/or therapeutic use of TDD for 1–12 days in 24 patients; this included one with RA. It was noted that the signs of inflammation around all the joints improved significantly within 3–4 days, only to return to pretreatment levels within 1 week after discontinuation of TDD. Despite a 50 percent reduction in serum gammaglobulins, the latex titer did not change nor was there a change in the absolute peripheral lymphocyte count.

Wegelius et al.[35] performed TDD for 3–7 days in 5 patients with RA and 1 patient with juvenile rheumatoid arthritis (JRA). The immediate clinical response was felt to be "good" in 3 patients and "fairly good" in 2 patients, with only the JRA patient failing to respond. Four of 6 patients demonstrated a prolonged remission of symptoms for at least several weeks before relapsing. Again, it was noted that although there was a significant reduction in serum gammaglobulins, there was no change in the latex titer. In addition, no peripheral lymphopenia was noted. Following the clinical relapse in these patients, 5 of 6 patients had a beneficial response from cytotoxics (drug not specified). In conclusion, Wegelius et al.[35] suggested that the effect was caused by a reduction of immunocompetent cells rather than of circulating antibodies, and they proposed that extracorporeal irradiation of circulating thoracic duct lymphocytes be investigated as a future immunosuppressive method.

The results of extracorporeal irradiation of thoracic duct lymphocytes was reported by Edgren[36] in 2 patients with RA. After irradiation with 2800 rads, each bag of collected lymph was returned. The first patient underwent TDD for 14 days, with a total of 24 liters of lymph drained; 29 liters over 18 days were removed and reinfused in the second patient. Both the absolute lymphocyte count and the percentage of T cells were significantly reduced in both patients.

A reduced phytohemagglutinin (PHA) response, as measured by ^{131}I-deoxyuridine incorporation, was demonstrated in the returned lymphocytes in both patients, although this reduction could not be demonstrated in peripheral blood lymphocytes. This suggested that the reinfused cells did not remain in the circulation. In addition, radioactively labeled lymphocytes from the second patient were returned, with increased uptake noted only over the spleen.

Concomitant with this reduction of both lymphocyte number and function, clinical improvement was noted within the first days of therapy and continued throughout the treatment regimen with decreased joint symptoms as well as reduction in size of rheumatoid nodules. Both patients, however, eventually had a recurrence of their symptomatology after cessation of therapy.

In 1977, Paulus et al.[37] reported a series of 9 patients with seropositive, destructive RA treated with prolonged TDD (19–105 days, mean 53.4 days). This prolonged drainage was accomplished by returning the cell-free lymph to the venous circulation, which thus avoids protein depletion. Total number of cells drained ranged from 17×10^{10} to 111×10^{10}, with a mean of 46.1×10^{10} cells. Improvement in grip strength, duration of morning stiffness, and the number of tender joints improved significantly in all patients, although symptoms of active arthritis recurred within 2–12 weeks after cessation of drainage.

It was noted that after TDD, patients were more responsive to conventional therapy, including gold salts and nonsteroidal anti-inflammatory drugs (NSAIDs). In addition to measurements of clinical activity, evaluations of both cellular and humoral immune function and circulation studies of reinfused lymphocytes were conducted.

Absolute numbers of lymphocytes in both lymph and peripheral blood decreased during the first 4 weeks of TDD and then stabilized; they returned to baseline within 15 weeks after completion of TDD (Fig. 4-2). IgG and IgA immunoglobulins decreased during the first week and then stabilized, but no change was seen in IgM, C_3, or in RA latex titer.

Reinfusion of ^{51}Cr-labeled lymphocytes revealed a 10-fold increase in surface gamma counts over the spleen and liver, with only minimal increases over inflamed knees. In later thoracic duct collections, approximately 1 percent of the radioactivity was detected. Fifty percent was cell associated, which thus demonstrated, contrary to earlier studies, that there is some recirculation of lymphocytes from blood to lymph. When live ^{51}Cr-labeled lymphocytes were infused, a transient flare of symptoms occurred, which lasted 7–10 days. This was not seen when heat-killed cells were reinfused. In addition, some live-labeled cells were found in synovial tissue after infusion; this suggests a role for some of the lymphocytes drained from the thoracic duct that were involved in the production and maintenance of the inflammation associated with RA.

TDD also significantly suppressed cell-mediated immunity, as demonstrated by prolonged homologous skin-graft survival and decreased delayed hypersensitivity reactions to dinitrochlorobenzene (DNCB). TDD selectively suppressed some humoral antibody resonses but had no effect on inflammatory responses to chemical or mechanical irritants. Interestingly, later studies in one patient[38] with the most profound immunosuppression during TDD probably demonstrated immunologic tolerance, since two later skin grafts from the same donor as the original graft (D matches), and which were placed *after* the disease activity had flares and other immune responses had

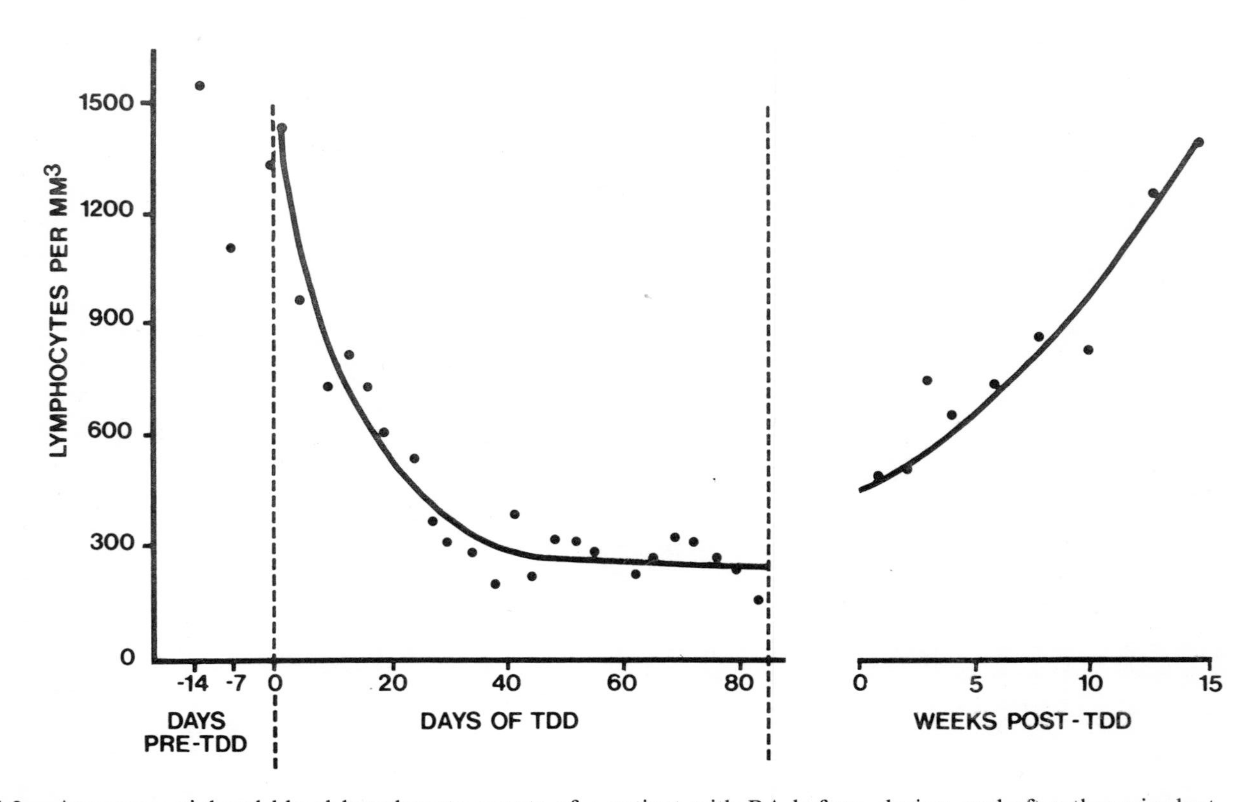

Fig. 4-2. Average peripheral blood lymphocyte counts of a patient with RA before, during, and after thoracic duct drainage. From Paulus HE, Machleder HI, Levine S, et al.: Lymphocyte involvement in rheumatoid arthritis. Arthritis Rheum 20:1249–1262, 1977. With permission.

returned to normal, survived without rejection, while a skin graft from a different donor was rejected.

TDD was not without complications. Two patients developed septicemia due to a batch of contaminated heparin; pleuropericarditis, thrombocytopenia, and neutropenia (associated with Felty's syndrome) each occurred in 1 patient.

This hallmark study by Paulus et al.[38] did not offer a new, important therapeutic modality for severe RA; TDD is far too costly, resource consuming, and transiently effective to be applied to the general population. The study did, however, offer significant insights into the role of the immune system and, particularly, lymphocytes in the inflammatory process of RA, as well as providing a scientific basis for both apheresis and total lymphoid irradiation, potentially promising therapeutic modalities. Although there appeared to be greater symptomatic and clinical responses with longer drainage times, recurrence of disease activity after cessation of TDD suggests that either some disease-committed cells may not circulate (perhaps sequestered in lymph nodes, spleen, or synovium), or that an insufficient number of cells were removed.

Apheresis

As noted earlier, attempts at treating RA with immunomodulation have predominantly involved the use of cytotoxic drugs. Although effective in certain instances, there is significant toxicity associated with the use of these drugs. Alternative methods have included techniques that attempted physically to remove either soluble plasma factors, which may be involved in the initiation or perpetuation of immunologic reactivity, or to remove lymphocytes based on their proposed involvement in the immunological reactions, with the hopes that the same, or better clinical results could be achieved with less toxicity.

Apheresis, in its various forms, has been used in attempts to accomplish both of these means.

The term "apheresis" is derived from the Greek *aphairesis,* meaning removal and is defined as "Any procedure in which blood is withdrawn from a donor, a portion is separated and retained and the remainder is re-transfused into the donor." Thus, depending upon which portions or constituents are removed and which are returned, various forms of apheresis can be defined. Although apheresis may be used as a method of collection of certain blood components (e.g., platelet pheresis), only methods of therapeutic pheresis and their utilization in the treatment of RA will be discussed.

With some variations, all the types of aphereses are conducted in a similar manner. Vascular access is required, either by means of large peripheral veins, or a shunt or a fistula is created. Most aphereses presently use a continuous flow machine that (as in hemodialysis) requires a point of exit for whole blood and a point of return for red blood cells and the plasma components to be returned (Fig. 4-3).

PP is the selective removal of plasma from whole blood, with return of red blood cells, white blood cells, and platelets; this necessitates a replacement of both volume and plasma protein, usually given as either fresh frozen plasma (FFP) or albumin with crystalloid solution. Plasma volume is estimated to be 40 ml/kg of total body weight, and a plasma exchange of 1½ times the plasma volume (usually about 4 liters) will cause a reduction of an intravascular component by approximately 65 percent. There exists a loss of diminishing returns with larger exchanges. Fibrinogen, C_3, and immune complexes are removed more efficiently (75–85 percent) than predicted; electrolytes, uric acid, and selected proteins are removed less efficiently than predicted. Recovery rates for various constituents of plasma also occur at different, more complex rates.

Cryopheresis is a modification of PP. After separation of plasma from erythrocytes, a second filtration occurs, which removes components with a molecular weight above a given threshold (usually 100,000 daltons). These secondarily filtered components are then precipitated by a temperature-dependent process termed "cryogelation." The obvious advantages of this modification are a marked reduction in the requirement for plasma replacement as well as avoidance of the removal of other plasma factors (e.g., electrolytes, smaller proteins, etc.).

Although utilizing extracorporeal circulation to selectively remove components of blood is also the basis of lymphopheresis (leukopheresis), by

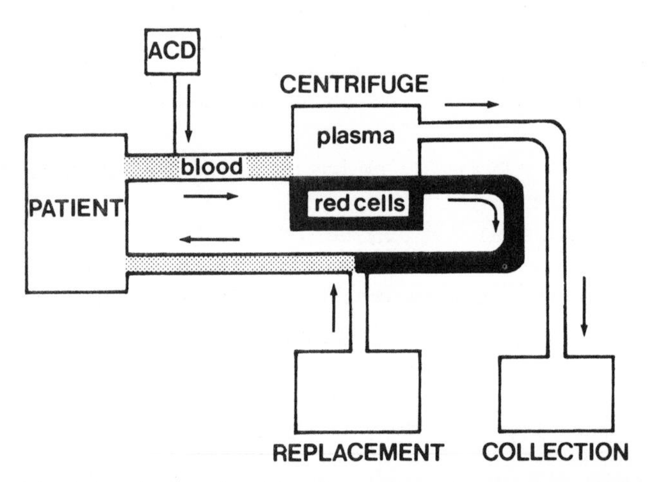

Fig. 4-3. Schematic of the plasmapheresis procedure. ACD = anticoagulant citrate dextrose solution. (From Linker C: Plasmapheresis in clinical medicine. West J Med 138:60–69, 1983. With permission.)

definition, the major component removed is lymphocytes with relatively small amounts of plasma; this is radically different in effect from that of pheresis. Removal of 5×10^9 lymphocytes per pheresis with thrice weekly treatments can result in absolute lymphopenia in 3 weeks. Again, the major advantage of lymphopheresis is the lack of need for plasma volume replacement, although there is an increased requirement for red blood cell (RBC) transfusion.

LPD essentially combines both PP (40 ml/kg exchange) and lymphopheresis (5×10^9 lymphocyte removal). Advantages include theoretic immunosuppressive activity from removal of both soluble plasma factors as well as lymphocytes. The need for plasma volume replacement and RBC transfusions are the disadvantages, however.

In 1963, Jaffe[39] demonstrated that PP (done by hand) could produce a decrease in rheumatoid factor titer with each pheresis treatment, although after five consecutive treatments, which removed approximately 600 ml of plasma, the rheumatoid factor returned to baseline following a 2-day rest period. No clinical improvement was noted following 8 days of pheresis over a 10-day period. Jones et al.[40] were the first to demonstrate clinical improvement in patients with collagen vascular disease when 4 of 8 patients with SLE were treated with removal of 5–8 liters of plasma weekly. All 4 patients who improved had high levels of circulating immune complexes (CIC) initially experienced a dramatic fall in the level of CIC as well as a fall in anticomplimentary activity (ACA), which was felt to suggest a possible unblocking of the reticuloendothelial clearance system (RES).

Wallace et al.[41] reported on the effectiveness of PP in 12 patients with severe RA in 1979. Eight patients were plasmapheresed 20 times over 11 weeks (removal of 40 ml/kg each pheresis), and 4 patients were lymphoplasmapheresed (LPP: 20 percent total circulating lymphocytes *and* 40 ml/kg each pheresis) an equal number of times. No differences were noted between the PR- and LPP-treated patients. Ten of 12 patients showed significant clinical improvement (6 of 8 PP and 4 of 4 LPP); this lasted 2 weeks to 8 months after completion of therapy. All 10 responders were on long-term administration (greater than 3 months) of gold or penicillamine. Of the 2 nonresponders, 1 was on Imuran and the other was on no disease-modifying agent.[42] Serological parameters (including CIC, erythrocyte sedimentation rate [ESR], IgG), although improved initially, returned to baseline values by the 20th pheresis. No changes were noted in the relative percentage of T and B lymphs. Toxicity was limited to anemia, thrombocytopenia (LPP only), and readily treated dysequilibrium syndrome. No electrolyte imbalance, hypocalcemia, or serious infection was observed. They concluded that "pheresis could be considered for those patients with RA who are underresponsive to long-acting agents but are able to remain on these agents."

This report caused considerable controversy, and Rothwell et al.[43] reported a controlled study of PP in 1980. Twenty patients with severe, progressive disease were hospitalized and given physiotherapy. Ten of these patients received (in addition) 6 phereses over 3 weeks with 30 ml/kg exchanges. Although immunochemical changes (IgG, C3, C4) were noted in the pheresis group, no statistically significant differences in clinical parameters were found. Objections were raised to this study because of the short course of therapy and because only 3 of 10 in the pheresis group were on either gold or penicillamine.

Two other studies reported successful outcomes using PP for synovitis (Dequeker et al.[44]) and for rheumatiod vasculitis (Scott et al.[45]); and Wallace et al.,[42] in a review of aspheresis, reported on an expanded series of patients from their original report.[41] In addition to a larger number of patients, most patients received a maintenance course, which consisted of 3 treatments in 1 week every 6 weeks or 6 treatments over a 2-week period. Each of these studies suffered from a lack of controls, small study size, and the lack of development of a standardized pheresis regimen regarding number of treatments and volume of plasma removed.

A controlled, double-blind study of LPP versus sham pheresis was reported by Wallace et al.[46] Fourteen patients were randomized to receive either 9 LPP (40 ml/kg and 5×10^9 lymphocytes) over 3 weeks or to receive 9 sham phereses. All patients were seropositive with erosive changes, and all were on disease remittive agents or cytotoxic drugs for at least 1 year; they remained on those drugs throughout the course of therapy. All patients were treated as outpatients. Toxicity was limited to transient dysequilibrium syndrome and a need for red cell transfusions in 4 patients. Two patients required placement of a fistula for venous access.

Assessment of Ritchie Index and self-assessment improved significantly in the LPP group. Ritchie Index alone improved in the sham group, but the difference in improvement (LPP versus sham) was also significant. Comparisons between LPP and sham groups approached significance in grip strength and morning stiffness. Laboratory parameters demonstrated reductions of absolute lymphocyte count, Westergren sedimentation rate, circulating immune complexes, and C3, IgG, IgM, IgA, and other protein constituents.

Although definitive conclusions could not be drawn from this study, because of its small sample size, several points raised are worthy of note: (1) short-term, high-frequency LPP is of temporary benefit in refractory RA, (2) a removal of greater than 5×10^9 lymphocytes for each procedure are required to reliably produce an absolute lymphopenia, and (3) concurrent therapy with disease remittive agents or cytotoxic drugs are necessary to prevent antibody rebound.

Even though side effects reported with PP were rare, the requirements for replacement of plasma volume are expensive and costly. In an attempt to accomplish the same therapeutic effect (by removal of certain plasma constituents) more selectively, and without requiring extensive volume replacement, a pheresis technique involving cryogelation (as described above) was developed. Krakauer et al.[47] reported the use of this technique for removal of large plasma proteins in a single patient. The patient underwent cryopheresis twice a week for 72 days, with an average filtration of 3–4 liters of plasma. A striking clinical response was noted, which was further amplified by the reinstitution of methotrexate, 10 mg/wk on day 40. CICs fell to 25 percent of their initial value, and analysis of the precipitate demonstrated immune complexes, immunoglobulins, C3, C4, rheumatoid factor, albumin, and fibrinogen. Serum albumin was noted to fall from 3.7 g% to 3.0g% after 12 treatments, and subsequent phereses included the administration of 500 cc of 5 percent human albumin after each pheresis.

In an abstract given at the 1982 Pan American Meetings,[47a] the data on 11 patients from multiple centers were presented. Of the 11 patients, all had significantly decreased CICs and 5 had decreased rheumatoid factor. Eight of the 11 had decreased Ritchie Index, 50-foot walking time, and sedimentation rate; 7 had total PIP circumference decreased. Complications included blood loss in 2 patients due to clotting at the filter and 1 case each of transient hypotension and soft tissue infection of the venous access site.

Five cases from a single center were more recently collected.[46] Each of these patients had undergone and responded favorably to LPP, with improvement in clinical parameters lasting 2–8 months. At the time of relapse, these patients received selective cryopheresis 9 times over 3 weeks, with removal of macromolecules greater than 100,000 daltons in size. Four of 5 patients clinically improved, as measured by the Ritchie Index and morning stiffness. All patients were on disease remittive agents or cytotoxic drugs. No plasma replacement was required. Cryofiltration of 40 cc/kg was found to be 70 percent as effective as PP in removing large plasma proteins. Decreases in IgG, IgA, and rheumatoid factor were noted. Interestingly, no decrease in IgM (which is decreased to the greatest extent with PP) was noted, and a decreased T-helper to T-suppressor ratio was found. This technique remains too untested to draw any significant conclusions.

Lymphopheresis (leukopheresis), although frequently involving the same technique and even equipment as PP, has an entirely different goal and approach to the treatment of rheumatoid arthritis. With lymphopheresis, an attempt is made to significantly reduce the total circulating lymphocyte pool by physical means. Lymphopheresis shares this approach with thoracic duct drainage and total lymphoid irradiation.

Tenenbaum et al.[48] treated 2 patients with severe unresponsive RA with lymphopheresis. One patient received 19 treatments over 6½ weeks; the second received 18 treatments over 3½ weeks. Each treatment removed 1×10^9–2×10^9 lymphocytes. Total lymphocyte counts were reduced by 50 percent, but the relative proportion of T lymphs and B lymphs were unchanged. Both patients improved by clinical parameters and subjectively; but during a treatment-free interval of less than 1 month in 1 patient, joint count and articular index increased. Reinstitution of therapy resulted in modest further improvement. Following therapy, both patients were placed on cytotoxic drugs (one on AZA, 50 mg daily; one on CPA, 100 mg daily) with maintenance of clinical improvement over a 4-month follow-up period.

Karsh et al.[49] lymphopheresed 4 patients 2–3 times a week for 6 weeks, with an average removal of 7.3×10^9 lymphs for each treatment. Three of 4 had prolonged lymphopenia, and all 4 had significant clinical improvement, which persisted after the 6-week treatment period; but each eventually had relapses, an average of 19 weeks after the onset of therapy. No cytotoxic or disease-modifying agents were used during this study.

The same group[50] conducted a randomized trial of 12 patients, with 6 receiving lymphopheresis 2–3 times a week for 5 weeks. All treated patients developed lymphopenia, and a significant dimunition of IgM was also noted in the treated group versus controls ($P<0.05$). Rheumatoid factor, other immunoglobulins and albumin did not change significantly. Clinical improvement, as measured by the number of active and swollen joints was greater in treated patients than in controls ($P<0.05$). Although morning stiffness and a 50-foot walking time also showed greater improvement in treated patients, these did not reach statistical significance. The magnitude of clinical improvement within the treated group did not correlate with either absolute or percentage reduction in lymphocyte; nor did it correlate with changes in IgM.

An interesting aspect of this study was that control patients had a volume of plasma removed equivalent to that removed incidently during lymphopheresis, which allowed the authors to ascribe the clinical changes more directly to removal of lymphocytes than in previous studies.

Toxicity in all of the aforementioned studies was relatively limited to mild, rapidly reversible dysequilibrium syndrome, the need for venous access, the requirements of blood replacement that depended on the exact technique utilized; the major side effect noted was the significant cost to perform these procedures.

The mechanism of action of apheresis remains obscure. Lymphopheresis has been shown to be effective in reducing the absolute number of circulating lymphocytes without significantly changing concentrations of other plasma constituents (except possibly IgM). At the same time, PP is capable of significant reductions of plasma proteins, particularly circulating immune complexes and complement, without significantly altering the white blood cell populations, yet both techniques have been reported to be effective in inducing, at least temporarily, partial remissions in the activity of RA. LPP, combining both of these techniques, and more recently cryopheresis, which even more selectively removes plasma proteins, had also met with relatively equal initial success.

A simplistic explanation would suppose that changing the overall milieu in which RA occurs would result in a change of the manifestations of this disease, yet sham pheresis[46] did not result in statistically significant clinical improvement and suffers from an inability to justify the removal of either lymphocytes or plasma constituents as an effective therapeutic measure. Several authors[40,51,52] have suggested that removal of circulating immune complexes may "unblock" the RES, thus allowing the body's own clearance system to become operational and reduce or eliminate the effect on tissues by these immune complexes. This has yet to be documented in a satisfactory manner, although it currently remains an active area of research.

Others have suggested that removal of lymphokines from plasma reduces the inflammatory response that lymphocytes are capable of generating. This could explain how either the removal of plasma (and thus lymphokines, the "incitor") or the removal of lymphocytes ("the effector") could both produce similar clinical results. Comparisons of several studies have indicated that the concomitant use of disease remittive agents and/or cytotoxic drugs (all of which may significantly alter the immunological precipitation, response, and effect of inflammation) may significantly enhance the ability to induce clinical improvement in the inflammatory response of rheumatoid arthritis as well as prolonging the effects of apheresis.

No study has been able to demonstrate complete and permanent remission of RA as a result of therapy, but one must suspect that perhaps even more intensive therapy, akin to that of treating a malignancy, would be required to remove every last functional mediator (lymphocytes) and/or incitor (lymphokines). All of the studies of the various forms of apheresis suffer from a lack of uniformity in treatment plans. How often must how much plasma or how many lymphocytes be removed, over what period of time, with what concomitant therapy, and how many maintenance courses are required to consistently produce significant clinical effects? The answers to these questions are, as yet, unknown and widely disputed; until more information is available, the true cost–benefit ratio of these very expensive procedures will also remain unknown. Certainly, the studies of apheresis can aid in our understanding of the mechanisms involved in the pathogenesis of RA, and these techniques remain a valuable tool for the very selected patients in whom an inexorable, rapidly downhill course can be foreseen; they can also be used in carefully controlled, larger study population experiments. The cautions raised by each of the authors, as well as in numerous editorials,[53–57] however, must be closely adhered to if any rational decision regarding the utility of these procedures is to be determined.

Total Lymphoid Irradiation

The lack of sustained remissions in patients with RA who are treated with thoracic duct drainage and apheresis reduces their utility in the management of large populations with RA. The procedures are too time and cost consuming and would need to be repeated in order to provide a continuous level of symptomatic relief. As suggested by both Paulus[37] and Wegelius et al.,[35] patients treated with TDD appear to respond better to NSAID, gold salts, and cytotoxic therapy following this treatment. Apheresis combined with long-acting agents (gold salts, penicillamine, and cytotoxics) appears to produce more lengthy remissions. Because relapses after TDD and apheresis occur, despite both modalities that remove massive quantities of lymphocytes, it has been suggested that the lymphocytes are involved merely as effector cells rather than being involved in the pathogenesis and that their diversion and depletion only temporarily affect the mechanism by which the inflammation and destruction occur. An alternative hypothesis would suggest that not all immunocompetent lymphocytes circulate, and by diverting only those that do, relapse is a certain eventuality unless all involved lymphocytes are removed or rendered ineffective. This theory is analogous to the approach used in treating neoplastic disorders, where it is felt that if even one malignant cell remains, malignant recurrence is inevitable. This theory is particularly interesting in light of the usage of radiation therapy in the form of total lymphoid irradiation, which is modeled after the treatment for patients with Hodgkin's disease.

Fuks et al.[58] intensively studied lymphocyte populations and immune function in 26 patients with Hodgkin's disease who were treated with radiation and who were in continuous complete remission for 12–111 months. These 26 patients included 15 patients treated with total lymphoid irradiation (TLI) only; 5 patients treated with TLI and intravenous colloidal radioactive gold; 3 patients treated with TLI and nitrogen mustard procarbazine prednisons (MOPP); 2 patients treated with mantle irradiation only; and 1 patient treated with radiotherapy to the upper abdomen. All measurements were done (with the exception of pretreatment total lymphocyte counts and immediate postradiotherapy total lymphocyte counts) at the time of continuous complete remission, which varied from 12 to 111 months after radiotherapy.

Total lymphocyte counts, percentage of T and B lymphs, and monocytes in pretreatment-Hodgkin's patients were not significantly different from normal donors (2038 cells/mm versus 1640 cells/mm^3). Immediately posttherapy, the total lymphocyte count mean was 503 cells/mm. Although the group of 26 patients in continuous remission regained normal total numbers of lymphocytes, they had significant T lymphocytopenia and B- and null-cell lymphocytosis. These changes persisted as long as 8–10 years in some patients. Prior to therapy, Hodgkin's patients had impaired responses of peripheral lymphocytes to PHA, concanavalin A, and tetanus toxoid. One to 10 years after successful treatment, there was little recovery of these responses. Mixed lymphocyte reactions, normal in untreated patients, demonstrated marked impairment during the first 2 years posttherapy; they gradually returned to normal by 5 years posttherapy. Testing of primary delayed hypersensitivity to Dinitrochlorobenzene (DNCB) revealed that 15 of 17 patients who were initially sensitive were anergic at the completion of radiotherapy, but 9 of 15 regained their hypersensitivity response during the first year after treatment.

Fuks et al.[58] concluded that radiation therapy and, particularly, TLI in patients with Hodgkin's disease led to a sustained alteration of both number and function of circulating T cells; they also concluded that some of these changes persisted as long as 10 years posttherapy; this suggested that radiation therapy may provide a potent modality for the induction of long-term immunosuppression.

The earliest studies on the effects of TLI on animal models with collagen vascular diseases were performed on NZB/NZW F_1[36,59] and MRL/1[60] mice. NZB/NZW F_1 mice routinely and spontaneously develop an autoimmune disorder, similar to SLE, with antinuclear antibodies, antilymphocyte antibodies, positive Coombs test, and a fatal immune complex of glomerulonephritis that is associated with aberrations of the immune system, which includes T-cell suppressor defects and nonspecific B-cell activation. MRL/1 mice routinely develop an autoimmune disease characterized by massive T-cell proliferation, accompanied by splenomegaly and lymphadenopathy, as well as anti-S, and anti-ds DNA antibodies.

Kotzin and Strober[61] administered TLI to 5–7-month-old NZB/NZW mice with at least low-grade proteinuria; they also administered TLI to 7-month-old mice with advanced (3+–4+) proteinuria. In the younger group, significant reductions in the progression of proteinuria as well as increased survival times, compared to controls, were observed. In addition, decreases in levels of anti-DNA antibodies were also noted. In older animals, there was an increase in survival and improvement in proteinuria, compared to controls; but this latter regressed several months after therapy was completed. Slavin[59] also demonstrated improvement in proteinuria, prolonged survival time, and decreased antinuclear antibody titers in NZB/NZW F_1 mice treated at 9 months of age with TLI; but again it was noted that disease activity recurred after partial recovery from the immunosuppressive effects of TLI.

Finally, Theofilopoulos et al.[60] demonstrated improved survival and decreased incidence of glomerulonephritis when MRL/1 mice were treated with TLI at age 3 months (time of onset of clinically apparent disease). These changes were accompanied by a 100-fold reduction of nodal lymphocytes and a reduction in helper T-cell activity, compared to controls.

Two more recent studies[62,63] examined the use of TLI for therapy of induced arthritis in rats. Schurman et al.[62] compared TLI, paw radiation, TLI and paw radiation, and controls in rats with adjuvant arthritis induced *Mycobacterium butyricum* suspended in oil. Those animals treated with TLI alone demonstrated a decrease in joint inflammation at the conclusion of therapy, but after therapy arthritis scores returned to pretreatment levels. The combination of TLI and paw irradiation induced a significant decrease in arthritis scores that were sustained for at least 1 year; this led the authors to speculate that continued inflammation was dependent on peripheral process as well as centrally in major lymphocyte-producing organs.

McCune et al.[64] pretreated rats with paw radiation and TLI 7 days *prior* to immunization with type II collagen in incomplete Freund's adjuvant. This therapy delayed the onset and reduced the severity of the arthritis, as well as decreasing antibody response to collagen and causing impaired PHA responses compared to both sham-irradiated rats and controls. When TLI (without paw irradiation) was administered 2 weeks after collagen immunization, there was no effect on the clinical course or extent of the arthritis, although there was a diminished antibody response to collagen.

Unfortunately, the *Mycobacterium* and collagen/Freund's adjuvant models of arthritis do not closely parallel the clinical course of RA. Both models tend to single, monophasic episodes of severe arthritis, without spontaneous remissions, eventually progress to ankylosis accompanied by a resolution of the inflammatory process. In addition, treatment prior to the induction, or even the clinical manifestations of the arthritis, is not analogous to the problem faced when treating patients with progressive refractory RA. The findings of marked diminution of inflammatory reaction with pretreatment are consistent with earlier reports of prolonged skin allograft survival in rats[34] and development of apparent immunologic tolerance to skin allografts in a human subject when the initial graft was placed during the profound immunosuppressive phase of thoracic duct drainage.[38] These observations, coupled with the apparent greater efficacy of combined paw and lymphoid irradiation in rats, again suggest that the destruction/division/depletion of lymphocytes merely removes, temporarily, the effector cells of the inflammatory reaction or that all involved cells are not removed or destroyed during these processes (e.g., sequestration of cells). Despite these reservations, the promising therapeutic response to TLI led to three studies of lymphoid irradiation in the treatment of RA in humans.

Strober et al.[65] administered 4000 rads to subdiaphragmatic lymphoid tissues to 6 patients. All 6 patients manifested profound depression in the peripheral blood lymphocyte counts, which persisted for at least 6 months. Four of these 6 patients demonstrated significant clinical improvement that lasted at least 6 months, at which time direct follow-up visits were terminated. Three of these 4 patients also demonstrated a marked decrease in morning stiffness and functional improvement.

This study was designed as a feasibility study, and longer term follow-up was not provided; but the beneficial effects without serious short-term complications led to a second study[66] by the same group.

In this second study of 11 patients by the Stanford group, 2000 rads were administered to the "mantle field" over 2–3 weeks. Subdiaphragmatic lymphoid irradiation with a total dose of 2000 rads was then administered without an interval period. Clinical improvement was not noted until 1 month after completion of TLI, but 9 of 11 patients demonstrated profound improvement, with joint scores reaching their nadir at 6 months posttherapy; they remained at that level for the 18-month observation period (Table 4-4).[67] Three patients had transient flares in disease activity between 12 and 18 months posttherapy, but no long-term trend toward relapse was noted. One patient was discontinued from the study because of severe lassitude, and one was discontinued

Table 4-4
Clinical Changes After Total Lymphoid Irradiation

Patient number	Months after therapy	Measurement of clinical change*			
		Morning stiffness (%)	Joint tenderness (%)	Joint swelling (%)	Global composite score (%)*
1	15	−92	−65	−59	−45
2	18	−91	−95	−88	−70
3	15	−75	−44	−70	−40
4	14	−83	−74	−67	−39
5	12	−98	−76	−55	−76
6	11	−90	−64	−86	−72
7	11	−50	−73	−42	−46
8	11	0†	−51	−33†	+ 6†
9	6	−88	−84	−72	−55
10	5	−50	+45†	−19†	−20†
11	5	−75	−91	−95	−43
Percent change (all patients)‡		−72 ± 9.1	−61 ± 12	−49 ± 10.1	−45 ± 7.6
Percent change (patients 1–7,9,11)‡		−82 ± 5.1	−74 ± 5.5	−70 ± 6.1	−54 ± 5.3
Absolute score (all patients)‡§					
Before treatment		7.2 ± 1.3 (hr)	57 ± 10	49 ± 6.5	34 ± 1.9
After treatment		2.7 ± 1.2 (hr)¶	18 ± 12¶	14 ± 3.6¶	18 ± 2.6¶

From Kotzin BL, Strober S, Engleman EG, et al: Treatment of intractable rheumatoid arthritis with total lymphoid irradiation. N Engl J Med 305:969–976, 1981. With permission.

*Percent change in each category is calculated from comparison of the average of the two pretreatment scores with the average of the scores from the last two observations.

†Decrement <35 percent.

‡Mean ± S.E.

§Absolute score is the average of the two pretreatment scores or the average of the scores from the last two observations. The percent change in the mean absolute scores before and after treatment may not be equal to the mean percent change in score.

¶Significantly different from the score before treatment ($P<0.001$ by Student's t-test).

because of profound neutropenia (this patient was later found to have Felty's syndrome). Transient neutropenia, transient pericarditis, and single dermatome herpes zoster were seen in 2 patients each. One additional patient had an exacerbation of rheumatoid lung disease 3 months after TLI. Constitutional symptoms of nausea, anorexia, and fatigue were noted in all patients during therapy.

Significant changes in peripheral lymphocytes were noted, which lasted throughout the 18-month observation period; they included the following: markedly decreased absolute lymphocyte count; an increase in the Leu2 to Leu3 (suppressor-to-helper) T-cell subset ratio; and a sustained suppression of in vitro lymphocyte function as measured by PHA, concanavalin A, pokeweed mitogen response, and mixed lymphocyte reaction (MLR) reaction. Interestingly, the one patient who did not respond clinically to TLI did not acquire suppressor cells of pokeweed mitogen-induced immunoglobulin secretion and had no change in the suppressor-to-helper T-cell subset ratio.

These results, although dramatic, must be tempered by the lack of a prospective double-blind, controlled experimental design (which is currently underway by the same authors) and by slightly, although significant, different results achieved by Trentham and his group.[67]

In this latter study, 10 patients received 3000 rads delivered to each of three regions (mantle, para-aortic nodes and spleen, and pelvic nodes) over 3–3½ weeks, with 2-week rest periods between each regional treatment.

Improvement was noted in 8 of 10 patients, usually beginning in midtherapy; in most clinical parameters patients reached their maximal improvement between the end of therapy and 6 months posttherapy. Return of synovitis and increase in indicators of disease activity were noted within 1 year after treatment in the 6 patients who had long-term follow-up, although most remained somewhat improved from the pretherapy baseline.

Absolute lymphocyte counts paralleled the clinical course (Table 4-5),[67] but T-cell subset populations were not done serially. Functional tests of cellular immunoactivity demonstrated impairment during therapy, but it again returned to baseline; this parallels clinical activity.

Adverse effects included fatigue and xerostomia in almost all subjects; dental caries in 3 subjects; weight loss and diarrhea in 2 subjects each; and anemia, thrombocytopenia, cutaneous erythema, and nausea in 1 patient each.

Differences in the way in which the radiation was administered by Kotzin et al.[66] and Trentham et al.[67] (3 fields over 14 weeks versus 2 fields over 5 weeks) may be responsible for the differing long-term results that these two groups noted. Both groups report on extremely low incidence of serious and/or permanent adverse effects, similar to that seen with TLI therapy used for patients with Hodgkin's and non-Hodgkin's lymphoma.

Coleman et al.[63] reported the experience of the Stanford group in treating Hodgkin's disease over a 7½-year period. Of 680 patients, 8 developed leukemia. No cases of hematologic malignancy were reported in patients treated with radiotherapy alone (320 patients), although one instance was

Table 4-5
Pattern of Blood Lymphopenia*

Variable	Before irradiation	Mid-irradiation	End of irradiation	6 mo after irradiation	12 mo after irradiation
White cell count/mm^3($\times 10^{-3}$)	8.5 ± 1.0	4.2 ± 0.8‡	3.6 ± 0.3‡	5.4 ± 0.6	6.8 ± 0.9
Absolute lymphocyte count†	2565 ± 357	420 ± 10 ‡	469 ± 19 ‡	1252 ± 108‡	3158 ± 421

From Trentham DE, Belli JA, Anderson RJ, et al: Clinical and immunological effects of fractionated total lymphoid irradiation in refractory rheumatoid arthritis. N Engl J Med 305:976–982, 1981. With permission.

*A total of 10, 10, 10, nine, and six patients were assessed during the five periods, respectively. Mean hematocrits and polymorphonuclear-leukocyte, monocyte, and platelet counts did not change significantly during the study. Data are reported as means ± S.E.M.

†Normal, 1500 to 3000 per cubic millimeter. The percentage of T cells was normal (mean ± S.E.M., 57 ± 7) before irradiation in the first six patients tested on entry into the study, out lymphopenia prevented serial assessments.

‡Significantly decreased as compared with the mean count before irradiation ($P<0.01$).

seen in a patient treated with radiotherapy and colloidal gold. More recently, Armitage et al.[68] reported 5 cases of non-Hodgkin's lymphoid malignant neoplasms (NHLMs) in 242 patients initially treated for Hodgkin's disease. Two of these 5 patients had received only radiation therapy and had been in remission for 24 and 52 months prior to the development of NHLMs. After they reviewed the literature, they discovered 24 other cases of NHLMs following therapy for Hodgkin's disease, 2 of which received only radiation therapy.

In addition to hematologic malignancies, cardiac toxicity from mediastinal irradiation has also been recently reported.[69] Twenty-five patients with Hodgkin's disease, who were treated with mediastinal radiation through a single anteroposterior (AP) port (a technique no longer used) were investigated by noninvasive means. None of the patients had preexisting heart disease, and none received cytotoxic therapy. Patients were examined 5–15 years after completion of therapy. Only 4 of 25 patients were noted to be symptomatic, 3 of whom were later confirmed to have a restrictive cardiomyopathy. In addition, 12 of 25 had EKG abnormalities, left ventricular end-diastolic dimension was decreased in 50 percent, and pericardial effusion present in 9 patients. Other less common, asymptomatic abnormalities were noted.

Both the authors of this study and an accompanying editorial by Hancock[69a] noted that the single AP port technique and the failure to use a subcarinal block are significant differences from techniques presently used. Although there has been a lower incidence of cardiac toxicity with these new techniques, only short and intermediate term follow-up has been available. The late incidence of cardiac complications remains to be determined.

The unfortunate lessons learned following the treatment of ankylosing spondylitis with radiotherapy[70] and the late (greater than 10 years) incidence of leukemia in people exposed to the atomic bombs in Hiroshima and Nagasaki (the period from 11 to 20 years after exposure accounted for 36 percent of all cases of leukemia reported)[71] must weigh heavily on the use of potentially lethal therapy for nonmalignant disease processes. One would, therefore, express a voice of caution in the use of this promising form of treatment for RA. McCarty,[57] in an editorial accompanying the papers by the Stanford group[66] and the Boston group,[67] urges caution in the use of new technological advances to allow adequate scientific study *before* widespread use makes this impossible.

REFERENCES

1. Levin RH, Landy M, Frei E: The effect of 6-mercaptopurine on immune response in man. N Engl J Med 271:16–22, 1964

1a. Santos BW, Owens AH Jr, Senseu Greugeo LL: Effects of selected cytotoxic agents on antibody production in man; a preliminary report. Ann NY Acad Sci 114:404–423, 1964

2. Maibach HI, Epstein WL: Immunologic responses of healthy volunteers receiv-

ing azathioprine (Imuran). Int Arch Allergy Appl Immunol 27:102–109, 1965
3. Hersh EM, Carbone PP, Freireich EJ: Recovery of immune responsiveness after drug suppression in man. J Lab Clin Med 67:566–572, 1966
4. MacKay JR, Dwyer JM, Rowley MJ: Differing effects of azathioprine and cyclophosphamide on immune responses to Flagellin in man. Arthritis Rheum 16:455–460, 1973
5. Curtis JE, Sharp JT, Lidsky MD, et al.: Immune response of patients with rheumatoid arthritis during cyclophosphamide treatment. Arthritis Rheum 16:34–41, 1973
6. Fauci AS, Wolff SM, Johnson JS: Effect of cyclophosphamide upon the immune response in Wegener's Granulomatosis. N Engl J Med 27:1493–1496, 1971
6a. Townes AS, Sowa JM, Shulman LE: Controlled trial of cyclophosphamide in rheumatoid arthritis. Arthritis Rheum 19:563–573, 1976
7. Swanson MA, Schwartz RS: Immunosuppressive therapy: The relation between clinical response and immunologic competence. N Engl J Med 277:163–170, 1967
8. Mitchell MS, Wade ME, DeCont RC, et al.: Immunosuppressive effects of cytosine arabinoside and methotextrate in man. Ann Intern Med 70: 535–547, 1969
9. Hersh EM, Carbone PP, Wong VG, et al.: Inhibition of the primary immune response in man by antimetabolites. Cancer Res 25:997–1001, 1965
10. Folb PS, Trounce JR: Immunological aspects of candida infection complicating steroid and immunosuppressive drug therapy. Lancet 2:1112–1114, 1970
11. Strong JS, Barthelomew BA, Smyth CJ: Immunoresponsiveness of patients with rheumatoid arthritis receiving cyclophosphamide or gold salts. Ann Rheum Dis32:233–237, 1973
11a. Winkelstein A, Rube FL, Tolchin SF, et al.: Mechanisms of immunosuppression and effect of cyclophosphamide on responses to influenza immunization. J Lab Clin Med 83:504–510, 1974
12. Denman EJ, Denman AM, Greenwood BM, et al.: Failure of cytotoxic drugs to suppress immune responses of patients with rheumatoid arthritis. Ann Rheum Dis 29:220–231, 1970
13. Jarrett MP, Schiffman G, Barland P, et al.: Impaired response to pneumococcal vaccines in systemic lupus erythematosus. Arthritis Rheum 23:1287–1293, 1980
14. Levy J: Comparative effects of azathioprine and cyclophosphamide in the treatment of rheumatoid arthritis, in Rosenthal ME, Mausmann HC, (eds): Immunopharmacology. Baltimore, University Press, 1975
15. Ziegler JB, Hansen P, Cooper DA, et al.: Monitoring immune function during immunosuppressive therapy. Aust NZ J Med 6:136–141, 1976
16. Ryckewaert A, Kuntz D, Lermusiaux JL: Study of the changes in delayed immune reactivity on the skin in patients with polyarthritis treated with chlorambucil. Rev Rheumatol 38:759–764, 1971
17. Heine KM, Stobbe H, Klatt R, et al.: Lymphocyte transformation tests in patients under treatment with immunosuppressive drugs. Helv Medica Acta 35:140–145, 1970
18. Bontoox D, Kahan A, Brovilhet A, et al.: Effect and mode of action of chlorambucil in rheumatoid arthritis: The importance of the lymphoblast transformation test. Rev Europ Etudes Clin et Biol 16:166–172, 1971
19. Santos GA, Burke PS, Sousentowaen LL, et al.: Rationale for the use of cyclophosphamide as an immunosuppressant for marrow transplant in man, in Bertelli A, Monoco AP, (eds): Pharmacologic Treatment in Organ and Tissue Transplantation. Amsterdam, Excerpta Medica, 1970
20. Starzl TE, Putnam CW, Halgrimson CG, et al.: Cyclophosphamide and whole organ transplantation in human beings. Surg Gynecol Obstet 133:981–991, 1971
21. Hersh EM, Wong VG, Freireich EJ: Inhibition of the local inflammatory resonse in man by antimetabolites. Blood 27:38–48, 1966
22. Bunch TW, O'Duffy JD: Disease-modifying drugs for progressive rheumatoid arthritis. Mayo Clin Proc 55:161–179, 1980
23. Amor B, Meoy C: Chlorambucil in rheumatoid arthritis. Clin Rheum Dis 3:567–584, 1980

24. Steinberg AD, Decker JL: Immunoregulatory drugs, in McCarty DJ Jr, (ed): Arthritis and Allied Conditions. Philadelphia, Lea & Febiger, 1979
25. Davis JD, Moss HB, Turner RA: Cytotoxic agents in the treatment of rheumatoid arthritis. South Med J 71:58–64, 1978
26. Stojanovic I, Budincia M, Nikdic J: Duration of improvement of rheumatoid arthritis after good response to cyclophosphamide treatment. Scand J Rheumatol 7:1–2, 1978
27. Wilkens RF, Watson MA, Paxson CS: Low dose pulse methotrexate therapy in rheumatoid arthritis. J Rheum 7:501–505, 1980
27a. Williams HJ, Reading JC, Ward JR, et al: Compression of high and low dose cyclophosphamide therapy in rheumatoid arthritis. Arthritis Rheum 23:521–527, 1980
28. Groff GD, Shenbroger KN, Wilkiens S, et al.: Low dose oral methotextrate in rheumatoid arthritis: An uncontrolled trial and review of the literature. Semin Arthritis Rheum 12:333–347, 1983
29. Zachamach H, Gruavet E, Søgaard H: Liver in methotrexate-treated psoriatics: A re-evaluation. Acta Dermatol (Stockholm) 55:291–296, 1975
30. Gowans JDC, Arnold G, Kaplan MM, et al.: Long-term therapy of psoriatic and rheumatoid arthritis with oral methotextrate monitored by serial liver biopsies. Arthritis & Rheum 22: 615–616, 1979
31. Roenigk HHJ, Auerbach R, Bergfeld WF, et al.: A cooperative prospective study of the effects of chemotherapy of psoriasis on liver biopsies, in Psoriasis: Proceedings of the Secton International Symposium. Stanford, Stanford University Press, 1977
32. Nylors A, Poulsea H: Liver biopsies from psoriatics to methotrexate therapy. 2. Findings before and after methotrexate therapy in 88 patients: A blind study. Acta Pathol Microbiol Scand: Sect AE 4:262–270, 1976
33. Warin AP, Landells JW, Levene GM, et al.: A prospective study of the effects of weekly oral methotrexate on liver biopsy: Findings in severe psoriasis. Br J Dermatol 93:321–327, 1975
34. Dumont AE, Mayer DJ, Mulholland JH: The suppression of immunologic activity by diversion of thoracic duct lymph. Ann Surg 9:373–383, 1964
35. Wegelius O, Laine V, Lindström, et al.: Fistula of the thoracic duct as immunosuppressive treatment in rheumatoid arthritis. Acta Med Scand 187:539–544, 1970
36. Edgren J, Klockars M, Weber T, et al.: Extracorporeal irradiation of thoracic duct lymph as immunosuppressive treatment in rheumatoid arthritis. Scand J Rheumatol 5:108–112, 1976
37. Paulus HE, Machleder HI, Levine S, et al.: Lymphocyte involvement in rheumatoid arthritis. Arthritis Rheum 20:1249–1262, 1977
38. Paulus HE: Prolonged thoracic-duct drainage in rheumatoid arthritis and systemic lupus erythematosus. West J Med 4:309–324, 1979
39. Jaffe IA: Comparison of the effect of plasmapheresis and penicillamine on the level of circulating rheumatoid factor. Ann Rheum Dis 22:71–76, 1963
40. Jones JV, Bucknall RC, Cumming RH, et al.: Plasmapheresis in the management of acute systemic lupus erythematosus. Lancet 4:709–711, 1976
41. Wallace D, Goldfinger D, Gatti R, et al.: Plasmapheresis and lymphoplasmapheresis in the management of rheumatoid arthritis. Arthritis Rheum 22:703–710, 1979
42. Wallace DJ, Goldfinger D, Thompson-Breton R, et al.: Advances in the use of therapeutic pheresis for the management of rheumatic diseases. Sem Arthritis Rheum 2:81–91, 1980
43. Rothwell RS, Davis P, Gordon PA, et al.: A controlled study of plasma exchange in the treatment of severe rheumatoid arthritis. Arthritis Rheum 23:785–790, 1980
44. Dequeker J, Naesens M, Martens J, et al.: The effect of plasma exchange on synovitis in rheumatoid arthritis. Scand J Rheumatol 10:273–279, 1981
45. Scott DGI, Bacon PA, Bothamley JE, et al.: Plasma exchange in rheumatoid vasculitis. J Rheumatol 8:433–439, 1981
46. Wallace DJ, Goldfinger D, Thompson-Breton R, et al.: "The current status of therapeutic apheresis in the management

of rheumatoid arthritis" in Ther apheresis and plasma perfusion; NY, Alan R. Lios, 1982
47. Krakauer RS, Asanuma Y, Zawicki I, et al.: Circulating immune complexes in rheumatoid arthritis: Selective removal by cryogelation with membrane filtration. Arch Intern Med 142:395–397, 1982
47a. Krakauer R, Jones JV, Smith J, et al.: Continuous flow cryopheresis in Rheumatoid Arthritis. Arthritis Rheum 25(suppl):S65, 1982 (abstract)
48. Tenenbaum J, Murray B, Urowitz EC, et al.: Leucapheresis in severe rheumatoid arthritis. Ann Rheum Dis 38:40–44, 1979
48a. Wallace D, Goldfinger D, Lowe C, et al.: A double-blind, controlled study of lymphoplasmapheresis versus sham aspheresis in rheumatoid arthritis. N Engl J Med 23:1406–1410, 1982
49. Karsh J, Wright, Klippel JH, et al.: Lymphocyte depletion by continuous flow cell centrifugation in rheumatoid arthritis. Arthritis Rheum 22:1055–1059, 1979
50. Karsh J, Klippel JH, Plotz PH, et al.: Lymphapheresis in rheumatoid arthritis. Arthritis Rheum 24:867–873, 1981
51. Hamburger MI, Gerardi EN, Fields TR, et al.: Lymphoplasmapheresis and reticuloendothelial system (RES) Fc receptor function in rheumatoid arthritis. Clin Res (Abstract) #246, S98, 1982
52. Hughes G, Ryan PJF: Plasma exchange. Ann Rheum Dis 39:95–96, 1980
53. Berkman E: Issues in therapeutic apheresis. N Engl J Med 306:1418–1420, 1982
54. Klein HG: Therapeutic plasma exchange: A healthy dose of skepticism. West J Med 138:92–94, 1983
55. Russell AS, Davis P, Percy JS: Plasma exchange in rheumatoid arthritis J Rheumatol 8:364–366, 1981
56. Arthritis Foundation and the American Rheumatism Association on Plasmapheresis in Rheumatic Diseases. February, 1981.
57. McCarty DJ: Treating intractable rheumatoid arthritis. N Engl J Med 305:1009–1010, 1981
58. Fuks Z, Strober S, Bobrove AM, et al.: Long term effects of radiation on T and B lymphocytes in peripheral blood of patients with Hodgkin's disease. J Clin Invest 58:803–814, 1976
59. Slavin S: Successful treatment of autoimmune disease in (HZB/HZW)F_1 female mice by using fractionated total lymphoid irradiation. Proc Natl Acad Sci USA 76:5274–5276, 1979
60. Theofilopoulos AN, Balderas R, Shawler DL, et al.: Inhibition of T cell proliferation of SLE-like syndrome of MRL/1 mice by whole body or total lymphoid irradiation. J Immunol 125:2137–2142, 1980
61. Kotzin BI, Strober S: Reversal of NZB/NZW disease with total lymphoid irradiation. J Exp Med 150:371–378, 1979
62. Schurman DJ, Hirshman HP, Strober S: Total lymphoid and local joint irradiation in the treatment of adjuvant arthritis. Arthritis Rheum 24:38–44, 1981
63. Coleman CN, Williams CJ, Flint A, et al.: Hematologic neoplasia in patients treated for Hodgkin's disease. N Engl J Med 297:1249–1252, 1977
64. McCune WJ, Buckley JA, Belli JA, et al.: Immunosuppression by fractionated total lymphoid irradiation in collagen arthritis. Arthritis Rheum 25:532–539, 1982
65. Strober S, Kotzin BL, Hoppe RT, et al.: The treatment of intractable rheumatoid arthritis with lymphoid irradiation. Int J Radiat Oncol Biol Phys 7:1–8, 1981
66. Kotzin BL, Strober S, Engleman EG, et al.: Treatment of intractable rheumatoid arthritis with total lymphoid irradiation. N Engl J Med 305:969–976, 1981
67. Trentham DE, Belli JA, Anderson RJ, et al.: Clinical and immunological effects of fractionated total lymphoid irradiation in refractory rheumatoid arthritis. N Engl J Med 305:976–982, 1981
68. Armitage JO, Dick FR, Goeken JA, et al.: Second lymphoid malignant neoplasms occuring in patients treated for Hodgkin's disease. Arch Intern Med 143:445–450, 1983
69. Gottdiener JS, Katin MJ, Borer JS, et al.: Late cardiac effects of therapeutic mediastinal irradiation. N Engl J Med 308:569–572, 1983
69a. Hancock EW: Heart disease after radiation. N Engl J Med 308:588–589, 1983
70. Brown WM Court, Doll R: Mortality from cancer and other causes after radiotherapy for ankylosing spondylitis. Br Med J 12:1327–1332, 1965

71. Bizzozero O Jr, Johnson KG, Ciocco A: Radiation-related leukemia in Hiroshima and Nagasaki, 1946–1964. I. Distribution, incidence and appearance time. N Engl J Med 274:1095–1101, 1966

72. Wallace DJ, Barnett EV, Nichols S: Immunologic dynamics in cryapheresis for rheumatoid arthritis. J Rheumatol (in press)

Muhammad A. Khan
Irving Kushner

5

Diagnosis of Ankylosing Spondylitis

Since the discovery of the association between HLA-B27 and ankylosing spondylitis (AS) in 1973,[1,2] there has been increased interest in AS and related diseases among physicians and scientists in general and, particularly, among rheumatologists. In addition to providing a major insight into the pathogenesis of AS, this discovery has also raised questions about our perceptions of the clinical picture and prevalence of this disease and about the appropriateness of existing diagnostic criteria.[3,4] It now appears likely that AS has a much wider clinical spectrum than is represented by its current definition. It has been suggested that AS may be far more common than has been previously recognized, and that it may occur in as much as 1 percent or more of the population, frequently in a relatively mild or subclinical form.[5,6] There has been a noteworthy increase in awareness of this disease; physicians are now thnking of and making this diagnosis in instances in which it might have been overlooked before. It is widely perceived that most rheumatologists and many radiologists have become much more competent in evaluation of roentgenography of sacroiliac joints than they had been in the past. Finally, typing for HLA-B27 is being employed as an aid in diagnosing this disease.[7]

DEFINITION OF ANKYLOSING SPONDYLITIS

AS is a chronic systemic inflammatory disorder of undetermined etiology that primarily affects the axial skeleton; sacroiliac joint involvement is the hallmark of the disease.[7a] In contrast to rheumatoid arthritis, in which articular involvement appears to be primarily synovial, joint involvement in AS appears to originate in bone, cartilage, and juxtaarticular ligaments as well

PROGRESS IN CLINICAL RHEUMATOLOGY VOL. I ISBN 0-8089-1646-7

as in synovium. A striking feature of the disease is the high frequency and rapidity of occurrence of fibrous and bony ankylosis, perhaps as a secondary consequence of the primary inflammatory process. AS is now considered to be the prototype of a group of diseases with which it shares many clinical, pathological, and roentgenographic features, as well as genetic susceptibility factors.[3,8–10] These disorders are frequently referred to collectively as *spondyloarthropathies* because of many shared features (Table 5-1). Patients with these diseases lack the nodules and IgM rheumatic factors that are characteristically associated with rheumatoid arthritis.

While the term "seronegative spondyloarthropathies" has been employed to refer to this group of diseases, the qualification "seronegative" appears to be unnecessary since there are no seropositive spondyloarthropathies. The spondyloarthropathies include AS, Reiter's disease, psoriatic arthropathy, enteropathic arthritis, a form of juvenile chronic polyarthritis, and possibly several other diseases.[3] AS may occur in association with these other disorders; but most patients have no evidence of these related diseases and are best classified as "idiopathic" or "primary" AS.

NATURAL HISTORY AND CLINICAL PICTURE

It is appropriate to review the natural history and clinical course of this disease before embarking on a discussion of laboratory aids to diagnosis, since AS is largely diagnosed, or at least initially suspected, on clinical grounds. The best diagnostic clues are offered by the patient's symptoms, the pattern and distribution of joint involvement, and the articular and extra-articular physical findings.[7a] We will emphasize clinical features early in the course of disease, when diagnosis is most difficult. The most common and characteristic early complaint is low back pain, usually beginning in early adulthood. Back pain is an extremely common symptom in the general population; while AS is not the most common cause of this symptom, it is an important cause of back pain and stiffness in young adults. Pain is initially

Table 5-1
Unifying Clinical and Laboratory Features of the Spondyloarthropathies

Radiographic sacroiliitis with or without accompanying spondylitis
Variable inflammatory arthritis of peripheral joints
Tendency for anterior ocular inflammation
Variable mucocutaneous lesions
Occasional aortitis
Increased familial incidence
Strong association with HLA-B27

felt primarily deep in the gluteal region, dull in character, difficult to localize, and insidious in onset. The pain can be quite severe at this early phase of the disease, it localizes in sacroiliac joints but is occasionally referred toward the iliac crest, greater trochanteric region, or down the dorsal thigh. Pain may be accentuated by coughing, sneezing, or other maneuvers that cause a sudden twist of the back. While the pain may be unilateral or intermittent at first, within a few months it usually becomes persistent and bilateral, and the lower lumbar area becomes stiff and painful. In some patients, pain in the lumbar area may be the initial symptom rather than the more typical buttock-ache.

Symptoms may be considerably milder in some patients. Pain may be absent or too mild to impel the patient to seek medical care.[11] Occasionally there may be only low back stiffness, fleeting muscle aches, or musculotendinous tender spots. Symptoms may be worsened on exposure to cold or dampness. Such a patient is often diagnosed as having "rheumatism," or "fibrositis," or, occasionally, even psychoneurosis. Back pain worsens after prolonged periods of inactivity and often causes considerable difficulty in getting out of bed. The patient may roll sideways out of the bed, trying not to flex or rotate the spine. At times the pain may awaken the patient from sleep. Some patients find it necessary to wake up a few times at night to exercise or move about for a few minutes before returning to bed. Another common early symptom, morning stiffness, may last up to 2 hours and tends to be eased by a hot shower, mild activity, or exercise.

With subsequent involvement of the thoracic spine (including costovertebral joints) and occurrence of enthesopathy at costosternal and manubriosternal joints, patients may experience chest pain accentuated on coughing or sneezing, which sometimes is characterized as "pleuritic."[12] At times chest pain mimics pericarditis or angina pectoris, and patients are mistakenly referred to cardiologists or chest specialists. Inability to expand the chest fully on inspiration may be noticed by some; mild-to-moderate reduction of chest expansion is often detectable in an early stage of AS and should not be considered a late physical finding.[13]

Sometimes the first symptom may result from involvement of girdle joints, i.e., hips and shoulders; these joints are involved at some stage of disease in as many as 35 percent of patients.[14] Hip joint involvement as the presenting manifestation is relatively more common when the disease begins in childhood or adolescence.[15,16] Hip involvement is usually insidious in onset and bilateral; it is potentially more crippling than involvement of any other joint.[14,17]

Involvement of peripheral joints other than hips and shoulders is relatively infrequent in primary AS; however, it may be the presenting feature in approximately 10 percent of patients.[18] Intermittent knee hydroarthrosis may occasionally be the presenting manifestation.[18] Involvement of temporomandibular joint with resultant pain and local tenderness may occur in approximately 10 percent of patients.[19] Involvement of these peripheral joints is usually not persistent or erosive, and it tends to resolve without any residual joint deformity in most patients.

PHYSICAL SIGNS

A thorough physical examination, particularly of the spine, is critical in making an early diagnosis of AS.[7a] There is often some limitation of motion of the lumbar spine, most easily recognized on hyperextension or lateral flexion. Direct pressure over the sacroiliac joints frequently elicits pain. In some patients pain may be elicited by certain maneuvers: flexion, abduction, and external rotation of the hips with the patient lying supine may cause pain in the sacroiliac joints, as may compression of the pelvis with the patient lying on his side. All these tests may be negative, however, since the sacroiliac joints are surrounded by strong ligaments, that allow only very minimal motion.[20]

Evaluation of lumbar spinal mobility cannot be carried out by gross evaluation of forward bending since good motion of hip joints can compensate for considerable loss of mobility in this region.[7a] Lumbar mobility can be reliably assessed by checking lateral flexion, hyperextension, or rotation; most physicians, however, evaluate lumbar mobility by employing the Schober test to detect limitation of forward flexion. This test is performed by marking on the skin that overlies in the spinous process of the fifth lumbar vertebra (usually at the level of the "dimples of Venus") and at another point 10 cm above in the midline. The patient is asked to bend the spine forward maximally without bending the knees. If the distance between the two points increases by 4 cm or less, decreased mobility of the lumbar spine is present.

Because of the presence of enthesopathy, important additional early physical findings (which are often overlooked) include tenderness over ischial tuberosities, greater trochanters, spinous proceses, costochondral and manubriosternal junctions, anterior–superior iliac spines and the iliac crest, and sometimes even over calcaneum, tibial tubercle, and pubic symphysis.[7a] Limited chest expansion in an individual with insidious onset of chronic low back pain who is without chest disease should strongly raise the possibility of AS. The normal chest expansion of 5 cm or greater is measured on maximal inspiration after maximal force expiration; this measurement is made at the fourth intercostal space in males or just below the breast in females.

As the disease progresses, the patient's entire spine becomes increasingly stiff and the patient loses normal posture. Lumbar lordosis gradually disappears, and the thoracic spine develops gentle kyphosis. With involvement of cervical spine, there is progressive limitation of neck motion; a forward stoop of the neck gradually develops. The chest becomes flattened and the abdomen becomes protuberant; breathing is primarily by diaphragmatic action. In advanced stages of the disease, when spinal mobility is restricted in all planes, the diagnosis is readily apparent because of the characteristic gait and posture and the way the patient sits or rises from the chair or examining table. By this stage of the disease, pain from spinal involvement diminishes and there is less morning stiffness; but some degree of inflammatory pain is usually present, even in advanced stages of the disease. Patients may have difficulty standing erect enough to permit the back of their heads to approach a wall against which their back is pressed (occiput to wall test). In extreme cases, the entire spine may be fused in a flexed position and the field of vision becomes limited; this makes it difficult for some patients to see where they are going as they walk.

PROBLEMS IN DIAGNOSIS

It is not difficult to make the diagnosis of AS in patients with such advanced, severe disease; x-ray confirmation is unequivocal and is usually redundant in the presence of such a clinical picture. The two major problems regarding the diagnosis of AS confronting physicians today are as follows:

1. How to make the diagnosis early, before the full-blown picture develops
2. How to make the diagnosis in patients with atypical disease, in whom the full-blown picture never develops.

ATYPICAL DISEASE

Historically, our concept of the clinical picture of AS has been based on patients with florid, unequivocal, and usually severe disease. Such considerations influenced the development of both the Rome and the New York criteria for diagnosing AS.[21,22] It has become apparent in the last decade that a number of B27-positive individuals, not previously recognized as having AS, manifest clinical features of spondyloarthropathy that are atypical or relatively mild compared to the classic, florid poker spine picture that, in the past, has constituted our concept of the clinical picture of AS.[5,6] As a result, our understanding of what ought to be encompassed in the diagnostic entity AS is undergoing evolution to include such patients with mild or atypical disease. To insist that patients meet the rigid classical criteria might be analogous to demanding that a patient manifest arthritis, butterfly rash, nephritis, pleurisy, and thrombocytopenia simultaneously before accepting the diagnosis of systemic lupus erythematosus.

There are now four groups of patients recognized who appear to manifest AS in an atypical manner or who do not fit our current criteria for AS but who perhaps ought to be regarded as having this disease. They are as follows: (1) children, (2) women, (3) individuals with characteristic signs and symptoms with absent or equivocal radiologic changes, and (4) radiologic changes of AS in essentially asymptomatic individuals.

Ankylosing Spondylitis in Children

It has become apparent in recent years that AS can begin in childhood, mostly in children after the age of 9 years, and it is 6 times more commonly seen in boys than in girls.[23] Back pain is often not the presenting complaint, the disease frequently presents as monarticular or pauci-articular arthritis; the hips and knees are the most frequently affected joints.[16,23] Less commonly, the patient may present with painful ankle or heel, polyarthritis, constitutional symptoms, severe back or neck pain, and very rarely even atlantoaxial subluxation.[16,23–25] A detailed family history can often be helpful; other family members may also suffer from AS or related spondyloarthropathies.

It may take some years before changes in the sacroiliac joints occur, which permits a definitive diagnosis of juvenile AS. Ansell[23] has observed that it takes a mean duration of 6.5 years from the onset of first symptoms of the disease to development of unequivocal roentgenographic evidence of sacroiliitis. Limitation of back motion takes even longer to develop (11–33 years in Ansell's series), and frequently back pain can be absent when limitation of spinal mobility is first noted. Pelvic roentgenography is not very helpful in making an early diagnosis of AS in children because the sacral epiphysis can be easily confused with sacroiliitis. Radionuclide scintigraphy is also not of much clinical help because the presence of epiphyses normally causes a high sacroiliac uptake. Not surprisingly, as among adult patients with AS, up to 90 percent of patients with juvenile AS possess HLA-B27.[16,23]

Ankylosing Spondylitis in Women

Several studies of clinical and roentgenographic features of the disease in women have recently been carried out and the results of these studies suggest that extensive ankylosis of the vertebral column is less common, and the clinical and roentgenographic features of the disease evolve more slowly than in men.[26–35] As a result, the diagnosis of AS is delayed for longer periods in women than in men.[29a,30] Joints of the extremities may be involved more often in women than in men with AS. Roentgenographic changes in the cervical spine appears to be more frequent in women, with relative sparing of thoracic and lumbar spine; however, there is controversy about these points.[26–28,31,34] Prognosis on the whole appears to be better in women than in men and there is said to be less pain. The B27 association with AS is as strong in females as in males. Recent data suggest that the male–female ratio among patients with AS may be close to 7:3 rather than 10:1, as reported previously.[26,36]

Symptoms and Signs With Normal X-rays

A number of individuals have been encountered, particularly in family studies, who may be regarded as having AS without radiographic evidence of sacroiliitis or spondylitis.[37,37a] Typically these patients have had many years of low back pain and stiffness. They may show tenderness over the sacroiliac joints or evidence of enthesopathy at other sites. Limitation of lumbar motion is often present. Such individuals, like their affected first-degree relative, are found to possess HLA-B27. Abnormalities on sacroiliac scintigraphy or computerized tomography have been found in some but not all of the small number of such patients studied.[38–42]

Sacroiliitis Without Symptoms and Signs

Similarly, family studies have revealed many B27-positive individuals who have roentgenographic evidence of sacroiliitis but who have no symptoms or signs.[29a,30] Strictly speaking, these patients should not be diagnosed as having AS but should be categorized as having "asymptomatic sacroiliitis." Nonetheless, it is difficult to imagine what disease process other than AS or a related spondyloarthropathy could cause such skeletal abnormalities. The prevalence of asymptomatic sacroiliitis in the general population is not known. This condition has been found to be equally distributed between the sexes in the families which have been investigated.[30]

Rarely, AS (with abnormal physical findings), syndesmophytes, and radiologic sacroiliitis, can occur in a patient who consistently denies ever having had any back pain or stiffness.[11]

PREVALENCE OF ANKYLOSING SPONDYLITIS

There is controversy about the true prevalence of AS among B27-positive individuals. Two often quoted American studies[5,6] of apparently "healthy" subjects who possess B27 have suggested that as many as 20–25 percent of B27-positive individuals exhibit roentgenographic features suggestive of sacroiliitis or spondylitis; the features are equally frequent in males and in females.[5] If one projects these figures to the population at large, as many as 1.5 percent of Americans might be suffering from at least subclinical or mild form of sacroiliitis or spondylitis. A similar study of Australian Caucasians, however, suggests that, at least in Australia, the disease is relatively much less prevalent.[43] Another recent study in Holland also failed to confirm the report of 20 percent frequency of sacroiliitis among B27-positive individuals in the general population.[30] Radiographic sacroiliitis was observed in only 2.2 percent of B27-positive individuals in Leiden, Holland, and AS (by the New York criteria) was present in 1.3 percent of B27 individuals.[30] In contrast, studies of families of randomly selected B27-positive patients with AS have revealed a 25 percent prevalence of sacroiliitis among B27-positive, first-degree relatives (16 times more common than in B27-positive persons in the general population); 47 percent of these relatives with sacroiliitis were asymptomatic and did not fulfill the New York criteria for AS.[29a]

These differences in reported prevalence in Caucasians of sacroiliitis and AS in various studies may result from different criteria for the diagnosis or from differences in interpretation of radiologic findings.[29a,30,36,44] It may be that studies that showed relatively high prevalence include many patients with relatively mild forms of AS. It is, of course, possible that geographic or regional differences play a role in these differences.

DIAGNOSTIC CRITERIA

Boland and Present in 1945 emphasized 11 features that may be helpful in making an early diagnosis of AS.[45] No internationally agreed on diagnostic standards, however, were established until 1961, when the first set of criteria was proposed at Rome.[21] These so-called "Rome Criteria" (Table 5-2) proposed that the diagnosis of AS should not be made unless x-rays show bilateral sacroiliitis and at least 1 of 5 clinical criteria was present. Although it was possible to make the diagnosis of AS without roentgenographic evidence of sacroiliitis when four of the five clinical criteria were present, bilateral sacroiliitis was recognized as the most important criterion.

In 1968, the diagnostic criteria were revised and graded at a meeting in New York (Table 5-3).[22] Radiological sacroiliitis was considered to be necessary for diagnosis. Moreover, with greater severity of sacroiliitis, the need for clinical evidence to support a diagnosis of AS was lessened so that a

Table 5-2.
Rome Criteria for Diagnosing Ankylosing Spondylitis*

Clinical criteria
Low back pain and stiffness for more than 3 months which is not relieved by rest
Pain and stiffness in the thoracic region
Limited motion in the lumbar spine
Limited chest expansion
History or evidence of iritis or its sequelae
Radiological criterion
X-ray showing bilateral sacroiliitis (excluding osteoarthritis of the sacroiliac joints)

*The diagnosis of AS can be made if 4 of the 5 clinical criteria are fulfilled or if the radiological criterion and 1 other criterion are fulfilled.

Table 5-3
New York Criteria for Diagnosis of Ankylosing Spondylitis

Diagnosis†
- Limitation of motion of the lumbar spine in all three planes: anterior flexion, lateral flexion and extension.
- History or the presence of pain at the dorsolumbar junction or in the lumbar spine.
- Limitation of chest expansion to 1 inch (2.5 cm) or less, measured at the level of the fourth intercostal space.

Grading of sacroiliac radiographs‡

Grade	
0 =	normal
1 =	suspicious changes
2 =	minimal abnormality, small localized areas with erosion or sclerosis, without alteration in joint width
3 =	unequivocal abnormality, moderate or advanced sacroiliitis with one or more of the following: erosions, evidence of sclerosis, widening, narrowing, or partial ankylosis
4 =	severe abnormality (total ankylosis)

*Definite ankylosing spondylitis can be diagnosed if there is grade 3 to 4 bilateral sacroiliitis with at least one clinical criterion, or if there is grade 3 to 4 unilateral or grade 2 bilateral sacroiliitis with clinical criterion 1, or with both clinical criteria 2 and 3.
†Probable ankylosing spondylitis can be diagnosed if there is grade 3 to 4 bilateral sacroiliitis with no clinical criteria.
‡The sacroiliac joints on either side should be graded separately.

patient with grade 3 or grade 4 bilateral sacroiliitis needed only 1 of the 3 clinical criteria to be diagnosed as having definite AS. There is not universal satisfaction with the New York criteria; some physicians still find it more useful to employ the Rome criteria, while others have pointed out the need for revision of these criteria once again.[4,30,46,47] For example, although grades 1–4 sacroiliitis have been defined, there is considerable interobserver variation in interpretation of sacroiliac x-rays,[44] especially regarding grade 2 sacroiliitis[29a,30]; interobserver variation in grade 3–4 sacroiliitis is considerably less. These criteria do not define the normal spinal range of motion. Another problem with the New York criteria is that it may not be possible to diagnose early disease because unequivocal evidence of bilateral sacroiliitis may require many months to develop in some patients with AS.[7,48–50]

Recently, Moll and Wright evaluated the New York criteria and found that thoracolumbar pain was too sensitive and too nonspecific a criterion, while limited chest and back mobility were both too insensitive and too specific.[4,46,47] These authors suggested that the criteria be numerically weighed.[4] More recently, van der Linden et al[30,50a] have evaluated the Rome as well as the New York criteria in first-degree relatives of AS probands, as well as in the general population. History or evidence of iritis or its sequelae (5th Clinical Criterion—Rome) and the New York Criterion of "history of the presence of pain at the dorso-lumbar junction or in the lumbar spine" were found to have no discriminating value. The same held true for the New York criteria combination of thoracolumbar or lumbar pain together with limitation of chest expansion below 2.5 cm. Based on the results of this study, van der Linden et al[50a,50b] have proposed a new set of criteria, which, when applied to families of AS patients, and in population studies were found to be more sensitive as well as more specific than the Rome and New York criteria. They feel that AS is present if there is radiologic evidence of sacroiliitis (grade 2 bilaterally or grade 3 unilaterally) in combination with at least one of the following criteria: (1) low back pain for more than 3 months, improving with exercise; (2) limitation of mobility of the lumbar spine in both the sagittal and frontal planes; or (3) limitation of chest expansion below 2.5 cm or, preferably, compared with normal values[47] corrected for age and sex.

A challenge to the applicability of these criteria is posed by individuals with radiologic sacroiliitis, without any clinical and/or radiographic evidence of spondylitis. In addition to this radiologic difference, such patients differ from classic AS in prevalence of HLA-B27; in various studies, between 40 and 70 percent of these patients are B27 positive.[30,51–54] Whether this syndrome ought to be regarded as a distinct clinical entity or merely as a forme fruste of AS is unclear. Perhaps the B27 allele serves as a severity factor in the spondyloarthropathies.[9] Should one reserve the term AS for patients with spinal involvement, as semantics dictates? We prefer to define AS (especially for clinical studies) as radiographic bilateral sacroiliitis, plus at least 2 of the 5 Rome clinical criteria, so that clinical evidence of spinal involvement is more firmly established.

LABORATORY AND RADIOGRAPHIC FEATURES

General Tests

Acute phase reactants are of only moderate value in the diagnosis of AS and are perhaps somewhat more helpful in following the course of disease on therapy.[55–58] The best studied indicators of the acute-phase response have been the erythrocyte sedimentation rate (ESR) and the C-reactive protein (CRP). Reports of "elevated" or normal ESR are difficult to interpret in view of the uncertainty about the actual normal range for this determination. In general, the finding of an elevated ESR or CRP in a person with low back pain tends to support the likelihood of inflammatory disease (in this context, AS) and argues against the likelihood of mechanical etiology.[59,60] An elevated ESR is said to be seen in up to 75 percent of patients with active disease, especially in the early phase.[56–58] A normal ESR has been noted in patients with clinically active AS in the presence of elevated levels of serum CRP.[55–58] It may be that quantitative determinations of serum CRP levels will prove to be of greater value than ESR determination in the diagnosis and management of AS.[61]

Mild normocytic normochromic anemia may be present in 15 percent of patients.[56] A mild-to-moderate elevation of serum alkaline phosphatase is seen in some patients; this perhaps reflects the occurrence of bony erosions and osteitis in this disease.[56] Mild elevation of cerebrospinal fluid protein has been noticed in some patients, perhaps as a result of mild arachnoiditis.[62] In the uncommon patients with AS from whom synovial fluid has been aspirated, markedly distinctive features compared to other inflammatory arthropathies have not been found.[63]

Mild-to-moderate elevation of serum IgA and IgM have been observed in some patients with AS.[58,63–65] Serum complement levels are normal or elevated,[64] but elevated levels of breakdown products of complement components have been reported.[66] While some authors have detected circulating immune complexes in the serum of patients with AS, others have not confirmed these findings.[67–70] Tests for rheumatoid factor and antinuclear antibodies are negative.

Radiology

Conventional Roentgenography

The characteristic changes of AS are primarily seen in the axial skeleton, i.e., the sacroiliac joints, discovertabral, apophyseal, costovertebral, and costotransverse joints.[48,71–75] The earliest, most consistent, and most characteristic findings are seen in the sacroiliac joints.[48,71–75] Various methods have been used to examine radiologically the sacroiliac joints; none is ideal because of the complex configuration and individual variations of these joints.[71,76] Most physicians consider that a plain anteroposterior x-ray view of the pelvis[77] is adequate for screening for suspected sacroiliitis.[71] When equivocal changes are found in such studies, a repreat anteroposterior view with 25°–30° cephalad angulation of the radiographic tube is recommended.[71] While oblique views of the sacroiliac joints have frequently been employed, they are technically more difficult to obtain since slight differences in positioning the patient may make comparison between the two sides difficult.[71] In our experience, suspected sacroiliitis can be adequately screened with either standard anteroposterior views or anteroposterior angled views of the pelvis; oblique views of sacroiliac joints add little and tend to be misleading. In contrast to computerized tomography, conventional tomographic views of the pelvis seem to have little to recommend them in patients with sacroiliitis or with other forms of back pain, in view of the high dose of gonadal radiation administered.

The earliest changes in the sacroiliac joints consist of blurring of the subchondral bone plate, followed by erosions and sclerosis of the adjacent bone. Sacroiliitis is usually symmetrical; the changes in the synovial portion of the joint (i.e., the lower two-thirds of the joint) result from inflammatory chondritis and osteitis of the adjacent subchondral bone. Since the cartilage covering the iliac side of the joint is much thinner than that which covers the sacral side, erosions and subchondral sclerosis are typically seen first; they tend to be more prominent on the iliac side (Fig. 5-1). In the upper one-third of the sacroiliac joint, where the bones are held together by strong intra-articular ligaments, the inflammatory process may lead to similar roentgenographic abnormalities.

The erosions of the subchondral bone progress and can lead to "pseudo-widening" of the joint space. With time there is gradual fibrosis, calcification, interosseus bridging, and ossification. Erosions become less obvious, but subchondral sclerosis persists and becomes the most prominent radiologic feature. Ultimately, usually after several years, there may be complete bony ankylosis of the sacroiliac joints, with resolution of bony sclerosis.

Roentgenographic abnormalities at the disconvertebral junction, the apophyseal, costovertebral, and costotransverse joints, and other sites rarely occur without sacroiliac joint changes.[48,71–75] In early stages of the evolution of syndesmophytes, there is inflammation of the superficial layers of the annulus fibrosus with subsequent reactive sclerosis and erosions of the adjacent corners of the vertebral bodies; this leads to "squaring" of the vertebral

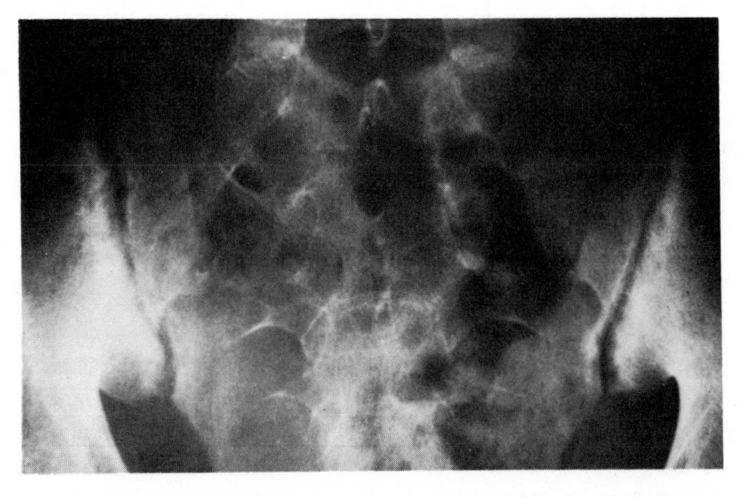

Fig.5-1. Anteroposterior pelvic radiograph showing bilateral sacroiliitis characterized by definite erosions and subchondral (marginal) sclerosis. These changes are more marked on the iliac side of the joint.

bodies. As the annulus fibrosus gradually ossifies, syndesmophytes form, which bridge the spaces between vertebrae. There are often concomitant inflammatory changes and ankylosis in the apophyseal joints; as more syndesmophytes form and as apophyseal joints ankylose, there is virtually complete fusion of the vertebral column (bamboo spine). Bony erosions and osteitis (whiskering) at sites of osseous attachment of tendons and ligaments are frequently seen, particularly at the ischial tuberosities, iliac crest, calcaneum, femoral trochanters, and spinous processes of the vertebrae.

At times, other diseases may be confused radiologically with AS.[77,78] In degenerative disc disease, changes are seen in discovertebral junctions and apophyseal joints, with adjacent osteophytes. Sacroiliac joints are usually normal or show only mild degenerative changes; erosions and subchondral sclerosis typical of sacroiliitis are absent. In rare patients, severe degenerative changes such as joint space narrowing, subchondral bone sclerosis, and bridging osteophytes in the lower part of the joint may erroneously suggest sacroiliitis. At times, the osteophytes seen in degenerative disc disease may be difficult to distinguish from the syndesmophytes of AS in patients who have concomitant degenerative disc disease at the time syndesmophytes are forming.

Ankylosing hyperostosis (Forestier's disease or diffuse idiopathic skeletal hyperostosis), usually seen in elderly individuals, is characterized by hyperostosis that affects the anterior longitudinal ligament and the skeletal attachment of tendons and ligaments.[79] While the ligamentous (upper) portion of the sacroiliac joint may become ossified (ankylosed) in this disease, the synovial (lower) portion is not affected but may show degenerative changes.[79a] Because there may be extensive spinal involvement in this disease, it may be confused with AS. As a rule, the two diseases are easily distinguishable because each has its own typical clinical and radiographic findings[79a] (Table 5-4). When degenerative changes of the sacroiliac joints occur in these patients, confusion with AS may occur.[79a] There is no association between ankylosing hyperostosis and HLA-B27; an earlier report of such an association[80] was not confirmed by subsequent studies.[81–83]

Miscellaneous conditions, which may be confused with AS because of sacroiliac joint involvement or syndesmophyte-like appearance of the spine, include Paget's disease,[84] fluorosis,[85] chondrocalcinosis,[86,87] and hypoparathyroidism.[88] Hyperparathyroidism can lead to irregularity of the sacroiliac joint surfaces, particularly on the iliac side, due to subchondral resorption and adjacent bony sclerosis; narrowing and ankylosis of the joint space do not occur.[89,90] Sacroiliac joint changes that suggest sacroiliitis and even complete fusion of the joints is seen in about one-third of paraplegics and quadriplegics.[91–93] Although these changes superficially resemble those seen in AS, they most likely do not result from an inflammatory process but may be a consequence of immobility.[91] These abnormalities appear to be related to the duration and level of disease.[91,93] Osteitis condensans ilii is an asympto-

Table 5-4
Differentiating Features of Ankylosing Hyperostosis and Ankylosing Spondylitis

	Ankylosing hyperostosis	Ankylosing spondylitis
Usual age at onset	>50 years	< 40 years
Kyphosis	±	+ +
↓ Spinal mobility	±	+ +
Pain	±	+ +
↓ Chest expansion	±	+ +
Roentgenography		
Hyperostosis	+ +	+
Apophyseal joints	—	+ +
Sacroiliac joints	—*	+ +
Anterior long. lig.	+ +	±
Syndesmophytes	—	+ +
HLA-B27 (whites)	8%	92%
HLA-B27 (blacks)	2%	50%

*The synovial part (lower two-thirds) is not affected, but the ligamentous (upper one-third) portion of the sacroiliac joint may become ossified. From Yagan R, Khan MA: Confusion of roentgenographic differential diagnosis between ankylosing hyperostosis (Forestier's disease) and ankylosing spendylitis. Clin Rheumatol 2:285–295, 1983. With permission.

matic roentgenographic finding characterized by a triangular area of dense sclerotic bone that affects the iliac bone and spares the sacroiliac joints.[94]

Radiologic changes identical to those seen in primary AS are seen in some patients with secondary AS, i.e., those with ulcerative colitis and Crohn's disease.[75] Spondylitis that accompanies psoriasis or Reiter's syndrome also demonstrates fundamentally similar roentgenographic features; however, there are usually subtle differences (Table 5-5)[7a,75] For example, in primary AS, syndesmophytes usually form in an ascending fashion, which initially forms in the lumbar spine and then appear in the thoracic and, ultimately, the cervical spine. Conversely, syndesmophyte formation in psoriatic spondylitis tends to be more random and usually does not have this ascending order of formation. Some physicians have used the term "marginal" to indicate the classical syndesmophyte seen in primary AS, i.e., syndesmophytes beginning at the angles of vertebral bodies. In contrast, patients with spondylitis in association with Reiter's syndrome and psoriasis tend to develop more bulky syndesmophytes that do not just extend from one vertebral angle to the other but start from the middle of one vertebral body and extend to the same area of the adjacent vertebral body. In the end, of course, differentiation of these diseases is based on accompanying clinical features rather than radiographic differences.

Table 5-5
Radiologic Changes in Spondylitis

	Group I*	Group II†
Spinal involvement	Symmetrical, ascending	Asymmetrical, random
Sacroiliitis	Symmetrical	Asymmetrical
Squaring of vertebral bodies	++	+
Syndesmophytes	++	+
Apophyseal joint involvement	++	+
Osteitis pubis	++	+
Hyperostosis	+	++
Paraspinal ossification	+	++

*Group I (a) Primary AS, (b) AS associated with chronic inflammatory bowel diseases
†Group II AS associated with (a) psoriasis, (b) Reiter's syndrome, (c) "reactive arthritis"

It has recently been suggested that sacroiliac joints may be completely spared in patients with advanced primary AS with "bamboo spine,"[95] as is occasionally the case in psoriatic spondylitis.[96] This must be extraordinarily rare. We have not yet observed complete sparing of sacroiliac joints in AS patients with advanced disease, despite our extensive study of over 300 patients. Dihlmann has reviewed axial skeletal x-rays of 2125 patients with AS; all eventually showed radiologic signs in the sacroiliac joints, although radiologic involvement in the vertebral column (such as "squaring" of vertebrae and syndesmophyte formation) preceded the occurrence of sacroiliac changes in 1 percent of patients.[48] In our experience, a few patients who were diagnosed as having AS elsewhere with "bamboo spine" and normal sacroiliac joints were found by us to have Forestier's disease.[79a] Subsequent tissue typing revealed absence of HLA-B27; this further strengthens our clinical diagnosis, since Forestier's disease has no association with B27.[79a,83]

Computerized Tomography

Computerized tomography (CT), introduced by Hounsfield in 1972,[97] has revolutionized the diagnostic accuracy and precision of many radiographic evaluations. CT images are produced by a computer-aided reconstruction of multiple radiographic projections in the axial plane as well as in the sagittal and coronal planes. Images can also be subsequently reconstructed for viewing from different angles and planes if necessary. However, as emphasized by Relman, it may not be advisable to accept such new techniques in an unqualified manner. He pointed out,[98] for example, that we clinicians should demand convincing evidence on costs and benefits before adopting this expensive new medical technology.

CT of the axial skeleton can be expected to be helpful because evaluation of pelvis and spine with plain radiographs can be quite difficult at times. This is, in part, due to the complex anatomy of articulations in this region; the curved oblique anatomic plane of the sacroiliac joints[76] and confusing shadows due to the overlying abdominal contents make interpretation of conventional radiography difficult. CT, because of its cross-sectional image format, is well suited for study of the axial skeleton; this includes the apophyseal joints and the outlines of the spinal canal.

Despite these theoretical virtues, the clinical role of CT in evaluation of sacroiliac joints and in the diagnosis of AS is not established. A recent study that compared conventional radiographs to computerized tomographic sections in an axial projection in patients with suspected sacroiliitis suggested that CT scanning may allow improved diagnosis and evaluation of sacroiliitis.[38,40] Borlaza et al.,[99] on the other hand, found no significant difference between plain radiography and computerized tomography when radiographs were interpreted by experienced radiologists. In studies we have carried out,[39,39a] CT of the sacroiliac joints did not reveal abnormalities when standard roentgenographs were normal. However, sacroiliac joints that showed only mild or equivocal abnormalities by standard radiography showed more obvious changes by CT. This issue remains to be resolved. In our view, it is only in rare patients that the superior resolving power of CT scanning is necessary for evaluation of sacroiliac joints (Fig. 5-2). In most instances, plain anteroposterior views interpreted by capable physicians can be expected to be adequate in determining whether sacroiliac joints are normal or abnormal. With further refinement in technical capabilities, however, it may be that this technique will assume an important role in early diagnosis of AS.

CT is of value in evaluation of cervical spine involvement and cauda equina syndrome[100] in patients with AS. Atlantoaxial subluxation, a rare complication of AS, is ordinarily detected by plain radiography of the cervical spine on lateral view in flexion, extension, and neutral positions. CT of cervical spine permits clearer evaluation of the subluxation as well as the dimensions of the spinal canal and the adjacent structures without the excessive radiation exposure that results from conventional tomographic views.

There is no question, however, about the usefulness of CT in diagnosis of back pain of a variety of other causes, which include herniated lumbar disc and spinal stenosis.[101–106] By using high-resolution CT, one can now visualize the spinal cord as well as its dural coverings, even without the use of the intrathecal injection of radiocontrast material. A resolution of 5-mm slice thickness seems to be the optimum choice for CT of the spine. Intervertebral disc protusions can now be quite easily seen with a high resolution CT scanner. In addition, the CT scan can anatomically locate a compressed nerve root, even at sites beyond the view of myelography.

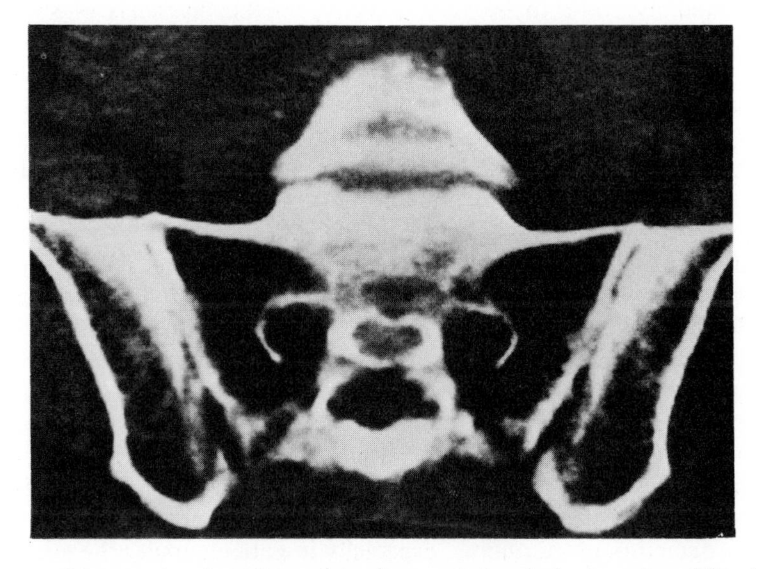

Fig. 5-2. CT scan showing bilateral erosions, subchondral sclerosis and focal areas of bony ankylosis. The scan was obtained on the GE 8800 scanner at 1-cm section intervals.

Radionuclide Scintigraphy

The other major recent technological advance in the field of radiology of joint diseases has been radionuclide scintigraphy.[107,108] Imaging with technetium-99m diphosphonate has been the technique employed by most authors in studies of patients with back pain. Distribution of radioisotopes is dependent on joint physiology (blood flow, bone metabolism, inflammation, etc.) as well as morphology. Techneticum phosphate compounds are bone-seeking radionuclides; their uptake into joint depends on blood flow, synovial vascularity, adsorption onto hydroxyapatite surfaces, and articular surface area. Increased uptake occurs at sites of inflammation, bone remodeling (both situations in which there is increased blood flow), and heterotopic bone formation. While changes on standard radiographs or CT scans show the bony consequences of previous inflammation, scintigraphic studies reveal current sites of inflammation since they reflect physiologic change.

Studies have been carried out that evaluate the usefulness of radionuclide scintigraphy of sacroiliac joints and spine in patients with early disease in whom sacroiliac roentgenographs show normal or equivocal changes. It was quickly learned that one cannot access sacroiliac joint uptake visually, because even normal sacroiliac joints show substantial radionuclide uptake. A number of quantitative methods were therefore developed; virtually all compared uptake over sacroiliac joints to sacral uptake. In some studies, cognizance was taken of the necessity of having age-matched or sex-matched controls, while other studies ignored this consideration.

Quantitative scintigraphy of sacroiliac joints with technetium-99m has been found by some to be very sensitive in the diagnosis of sacroiliitis associated with AS, psoriasis, Reiter's syndrome, Crohn's disease, and ulcerative colitis, but abnormal values have also been found in many cases of rheumatoid arthritis as well as in women with low back pain without evidence of sacroiliitis.[42,108–113] There is, however, considerable overlap between patients with sacroiliitis and normal controls as well as patients with metabolic bone disease or structural abnormalities of the low back.[39a,42,114,115] Furthermore, some have observed normal findings in patients with apparently unequivocal sacroiliitis, which leads to the conclusion that the technique is not very useful for early diagnosis of sacroiliitis.[39a,48,114–117] In our own studies, we employed a modified technique that permitted analysis of sacroiliac uptake in greater detail.[39,39a] We observed that there is a gradual decrease of sacroiliac uptake with advancing age in normal individuals and that uptake is greater in men than in women[39a] (Fig. 5-3). Abnormal findings were noted in a few patients with normal sacroiliac joints on plain film who were felt to have sacroiliitis on clinical grounds. All were over 30 years of age. Nonetheless, on balance these studies suggested that sacroiliac scintigraphy is not likely to be of value in early detection of sacroiliitis, especially in patients under the age of 30 in whom AS is most likely to be considered.[39a] In our view, it is unlikely that scintigraphy will be of significant diagnostic value in the absence of any further improvement in this method.

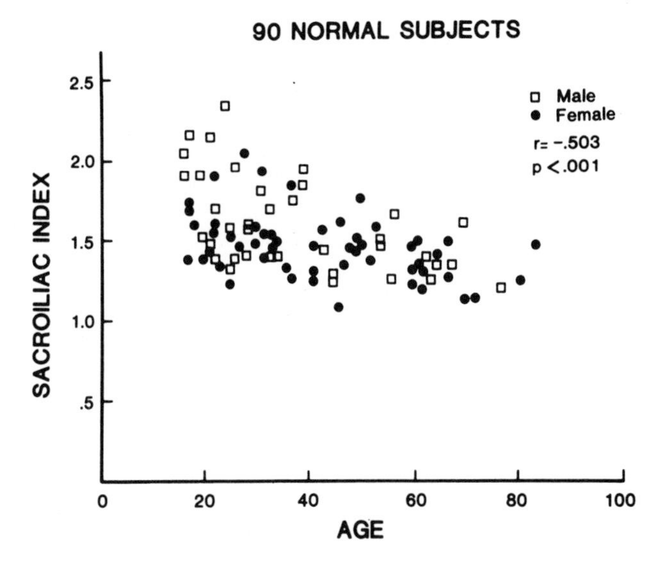

Fig. 5-3. Uptake of Tc-99m diphosphonate in the sacroiliac joints in 90 "normal" controls (37 males and 53 females) who had bone scintigrams for various reasons other than sacroiliitis[39a]. None had back pain; patients with skeletal metastases or disturbances of calcium and phosphorus metabolism were excluded. The sacroiliac index is a numerical representation of the sacroiliac uptake obtained by calculating the ratio of sacroiliac joint to sacrum uptake. With advancing age, sacroiliac index gradually declines ($p<0.001$).

Although not relevant to the diagnosis of AS, it seems appropriate to point out an instance in which scintigraphy may be of value in the management of patients with AS. A focal area of radionuclide uptake in the spine of a patient with longstanding AS who develops back or neck pain of recent onset, with or without a history of recent trauma, may indicate a fracture. Patients with AS are particularly prone to development of vertebral fractures with minimal trauma. Such fractures may not be readily obvious on plain roentgenography. In addition, quantitative scintigraphy is also quite useful in evaluation of patients with painful total hip prosthesis.[118,119]

Thermography

Thermography is a technique that records infrared radiation at the skin surface. It can be used to detect the abnormal body surface temperatures that reflect the increased blood flow to inflamed underlying tissues. A recent study found infrared thermography to be of little value in the diagnosis of early sacroiliitis.[120]

Nuclear Magnetic Resonance

Another noninvasive new tool, nuclear magnetic resonance (NMR), has great potential applications and has many advantages over CT.[121] Unlike CT, NMR does not involve radiation exposure; it is performed by application of magnetic fields to the tissues, and a computer reconstructs images of the spatial distribution of various nuclei. It is hoped that NMR may help in early detection of inflammatory as well as noninflammatory diseases of the back. No studies of its use in AS have been reported.

HLA-B27 Testing

The clinical usefulness of HLA-B27 typing in the diagnosis of AS has been the subject of some controversy.[7,50,122–125] In order to put this controversy in proper perspective, we will first review some technical aspects of B27 typing, evaluate how the results of B27 testing may influence our diagnostic conclusions (employing Bayes' theorem), and, finally, attempt to define the proper role of the test in clinical practice.

HLA typing gives results of high precision and accuracy. Several different well-characterized antisera, however, are needed for the detection of each HLA antigen because of the presence of cross-reactions.[126] For example, HLA-B27 belongs to a cross-reacting group that includes B7, Bw22, B40, and Bw42. An operationally monospecific antiserum against any of these antigens is very rare, and there has been only limited success in attempts to produce a useful truly monospecific anti-B27 antiserum.[127–129] When a reputable laboratory, therefore, wishes to test for B27, the recommended procedure has been to test for the other cross-reacting HLA antigens as well.[126]

As in the other common rheumatic diseases, the best diagnostic clues in AS are offered by the patient's symptoms, the pattern and distribution of joint involvement, the articular and extra-articular physical findings, and careful evaluation of x-rays as described above. Nevertheless, the value of specialized laboratory tests such as B27 typing in certain circumstances cannot be denied. Experienced clinicians with good clinical judgment have learned when to tolerate a certain degree of uncertainty about a diagnosis and when to order tests that permit them to minimize their uncertainty. It appears that B27 typing can, at times, accomplish this latter purpose.[7,122]

In order to evaluate the ability of B27 typing, or indeed any diagnostic test, to help in accepting or rejecting a diagnostic possibility, it is important first to define precisely the terms "sensitivity," "specificity," and "predictive value" of the test. Sensitivity is defined as the likelihood of a positive test result in a group of individuals with the disease, and specificity is defined as the likelihood of a negative test result in a group of individuals without the disease. A perfect test would always yield positive results in the presence of the disease (i.e., 100 percent sensitive) and negative results in the absence of the disease (i.e., 100 percent specific).

To ascertain the sensitivity and specificity of the B27 test, we analyzed the results obtained in our own studies of 140 white and 38 black patients with AS.[130–132] For comparison, findings in 54 white and 20 black patients with Reiter's syndrome are included.[7,133] The clinical diagnosis in each of these patients had been made before B27 testing and was not influenced by the test result. The frequency of B27 among our patients and controls is shown in Table 5-6. Most other investigators have obtained similar results, although differing values for the frequency of B27 among white patients with Reiter's syndrome have been reported; they range from 63 to 96 percent.[9,134–140] These wide variations may result from differences in diagnostic criteria.

The values for diseased individuals represent the sensitivity of the B27 test in American whites and blacks. Note that the sensitivity of this test differs for each disease and differs in the two racial groups within each disease. Because the frequency of B27 in the normal population is 8 percent among whites and 2 percent among blacks, the specificity of the B27 test (for both AS and Reiter's syndrome) is 92 percent in whites and 98 percent in blacks.[7] Since there is neither 100 percent specificity nor 100 percent sensitivity, B27 typing is not a perfect test for AS or Reiter's syndrome.

The usefulness of a test depends on the clinical setting in which it is performed. Tests are not done in a vacuum. A test that is very valuable in a particular clinical setting might be useless if performed on a random population. The predictive value of a test in a particular clinical setting depends on the pretest estimate that the disease is present. It reflects the magnitude of decrease in degree of uncertainty about the diagnosis, once the test results are known.[7] The same test may have great predictive value in one individual and little value in another; this depends on the a priori estimate of disease, which in turn is based on history, physical examination, and other laboratory results as well as on the physician's clinical skills.[7,122,141]

Two equations based on Bayes' theorem permit us to determine what our post-test estimate of the likelihood of the diagnosis ought to be in a given patient if the test is positive and what that estimate becomes if the test is negative.[7] In these equations and in subsequent figures and tables, the phrase "pre-test probability" of disease indicates the physician's estimate of the likelihood that a given patient has the disease, based on his or her clinical assessment, but before the test in question (in this case B27 typing) is done. "Post-test probability" of disease is the physician's new estimate of what the disease likelihood is, once the test result is known.

Table 5-6
Frequency of HLA-B27 in Patients and Controls (%)

	Ankylosing spondylitis	Reiter's syndrome	Normals
White	92	75	8
Black	50	40	2

If the test result is positive, the post-test likelihood that an individual actually has the disease is equal to

$$\frac{100}{1+\left(\frac{100\text{—\% pretest probability of disease}}{\text{\% pretest probability of disease}}\right)\left(\frac{100\text{—\% specificity}}{\text{\% sensitivity}}\right)}$$

If the test result is negative, the posttest likelihood of the diagnosis is

$$\frac{100}{1+\left(\frac{100\text{–\% pretest probability of disease}}{\text{\% pretest probability of disease}}\right)\left(\frac{\text{\% specificity}}{100\text{–\% sensitivity}}\right)}$$

The pre-test and post-test probabilities of AS in white persons with positive and negative B27 test results are depicted graphically in Figure 5-4. In this figure, numerical, rather than verbal, impressionistic estimates of disease probability are employed. Although physicians tend to use terms such as "likely," "pathognomonic," "classic," "consistent with," "possible," and "unlikely," there is marked variation in the interpretation of these terms by individual physicians.[142] Most physicians would not object to expressing their estimates in approximate numerical terms.

Figure 5-4 illustrates the usefulness of B27 typing as an aid to diagnosis by quantitation of the extent to which the degree of uncertainty is reduced after the test result is known and by illustration of how the predictive value (degree of diagnostic usefulness) of the test varies according to the physician's estimate of the pretest probability that a patient has the disease. The predictive value is obviously great when there is a great deal of pretest uncertainty (pretest probability about 0.5). In such a case, if the test result is positive, there is a 92 percent likelihood that the patient has the disease, an incremental gain of 42 percent. Ninety-two percent is an acceptable likelihood that the diagnosis is correct; although it does not provide 100 percent assurance, few tests do. If the test result is negative, there is only an 8 percent likelihood that the patient suffers from AS, i.e., the probability of no disease is 92 percent.

Even for the same patient, the pretest probability is likely to vary from one physician to another, in accordance with the physician's clinical experience and skills. An experienced physician with a particular interest in AS may be certain that the patient does or does not have AS after initial workup and will have little use for the B27 test. In contrast, another physician with less experience and less certainty about the diagnosis may regard this test as useful in the same patient. Such a physician may think the patient probably does not have AS but may be uncertain enough to feel that there is a 10

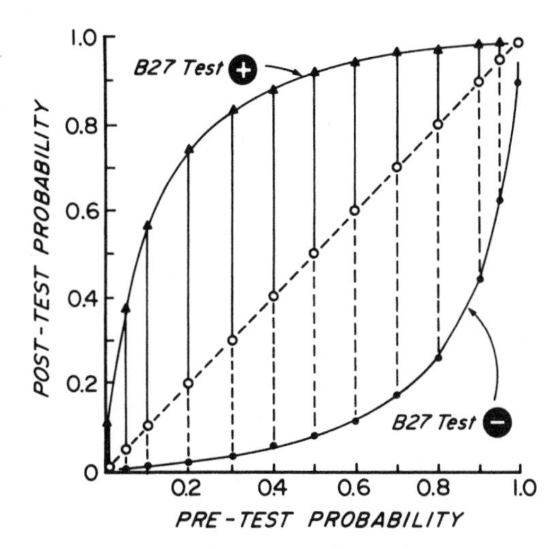

Fig. 5-4. Probability graph depicting the predictive value of HLA-B27 testing in ankylosing spondylitis in whites. The horizontal axis depicts the physician's estimate of the probability that a patient has the disease before the test is done (pre-test probability). The post-test probability is shown along the vertical axis. The vertical lines indicate the predictive values of the test at different assumed pre-test probabilities. The solid curved lines connect points that indicate post-test probability of disease, following positive (+) or negative (−) B27 test results. (From Khan MA, Khan MK: Diagnostic value of HLA-B27 testing in ankylosing spondylitis or Reiter's syndrome. Ann Intern Med 84:1–7, 1976. With permission.)

percent chance that AS may be present. The physician may regard that a negative test result is helpful, since this may virtually rule out the disease and allay his or her anxieties about missing the diagnosis. Of course, such relatively uncritical use of this test might lead to a false diagnosis of AS by such a physician if the test result is positive. For example, a positive test result in such a clinical situation (where the physician's pretest estimate of the likelihood of AS is 10 percent), simply indicates that there is a 56 percent likelihood that AS may be present; however, this likelihood is not high enough to make a confident diagnosis of AS.

Our delineation of Bayesian analysis here is not to be taken to mean that we feel physicians ought to employ such graphs routinely in clinical decision making. We tend to agree with the observation of Eddy and Clanton[143] that the notorious inability of human beings to manipulate probabilities in their heads makes it very difficult to use Bayes' theorem in a routine manner. Rather, our goal is to provide insight into the true significance of positive and negative test results in different clinical situations.

In the case of AS, most patients can be readily diagnosed clinically without the B27 test. In circumstances in which a clinical suspicion of AS that presents in an unusual or an atypical manner is raised and in adolescents, in whom the earliest radiologic changes of sacroiliitis may be difficult to recognize with certainty, detection of B27 can be helpful in supporting the diagnosis. But the test is useful only in a situation in which a patient exhibits symptoms and signs suggestive of but not diagnostic of AS. The test is of little or no use if the physician is already pretty certain that the patient does or does not have the disease. The B27 test is obviously much less useful when the pretest probability of AS is close to zero or close to 100 percent because of the minimal incremental gains for "confirming" or "precluding" the initial clinical suspicion of AS.

It cannot be overemphasized that the presence of B27 does not establish the diagnosis of any particular disease; it merely provides support for the diagnosis of AS and related spondyloarthropathies.[7,122] All of these diseases show associations with B27; the differentiation between these diseases is purely on a clinical basis.[9,10] Conversely, the absence of B27 does not exclude these diseases; all these diseases may occur in individuals who lack B27.[9,10,131]

Although B27 typing can identify individuals at increased risk for developing AS or related spondyloarthropathies, such identification is of limited clinical value at this time since no effective means of prevention are available. Furthermore, these diseases never develop in the majority of B27-positive individuals. It is thus important that clinicians avoid inducing undue anxiety in healthy B27-positive individuals. If effective means of prevention become available in the future, B27 ascertainment at an early stage might prove useful for the identification of individuals at risk.

Some clinicians might argue that when a patient's medical history and physical examination are somewhat suggestive of AS but there is no roentgenographic evidence of bilateral sacroiliitis, it might be sufficient to treat the patient with nonsteroidal anti-inflammatory drugs and physical therapy and to follow the clinical response without doing the B27 test. In such a clinical situation, however, the expected clinical value of the information obtained from the B27 test exceeds the risk and cost of obtaining it, because the information can result in a substantial change in probabilities; this produces a change in the preferred treatment.[7] Moreover, with early disease recognition, the patient will be spared the uncertainty of a provisional and perhaps incorrect diagnosis. Although no cure has yet been found for AS, accurate and early diagnosis is believed to be important in its proper management. Early diagnosis is critical because it facilitates early initiation of patient education and appropriate measures to prevent deformity, which thus potentially improves the patient's outcome. Nonsteroidal anti-inflammatory drugs are quite effective in relieving symptoms, and there is tentative evidence that one of these drugs, phenylbutazone, may alter the course of disease.[144] A major additional advantage of arriving at a correct diagnosis is that risky, ineffective, or inappropriate diagnostic and therapeutic procedures may be avoided.

The significant association between AS and B27 holds true in all racial groups studied thus far, but the percentage of B27 positivity in AS patients and the frequency of B27 in the general population differ in various racial groups.[9,10,131] As a result, the predictive value of a positive B27 test is slightly greater in most other racial groups than in European Caucasoids, but the

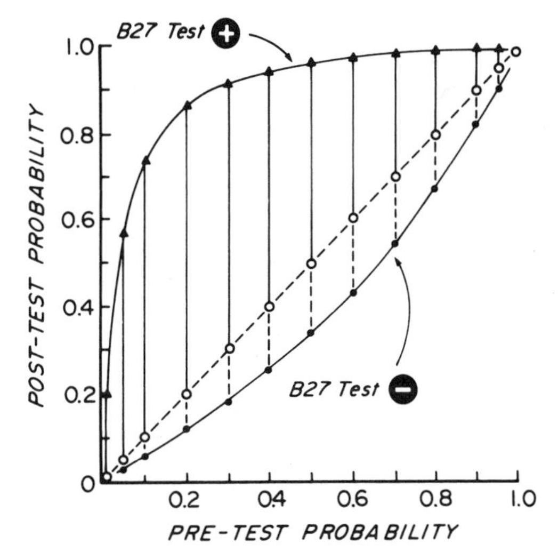

Fig. 5-5. Probability graph describing the predictive value of HLA-B27 testing in ankylosing spondylitis in blacks. The horizontal axis depicts the physician's estimate of the probability that a patient has the disease before the test is done (pre-test probability). The post-test probability is shown along the vertical axis. The vertical lines indicate the predictive values of the test at different assumed pre-test probabilities. The solid curved lines connect points that indicate post-test probability of disease, following positive (+) or negative (−) B27 test results. (From Khan MA, Khan MK: Diagnostic value of HLA-B27 testing in ankylosing spondylitis or Reiter's syndrome. Ann Intern Med 84:1–7, 1976. With permission.)

predictive value of a negative test result is substantially less.[7,122,123] For example, if the B27 test is done in a black patient with an a priori estimate of likelihood of AS of 50 percent, a positive test result would raise that likelihood to 94 percent (Fig. 5-5), while a negative test result would lower that likelihood only a small amount, to 34 percent. Similarly, the predictive value of B27 testing in Reiter's disease differs in the two races (Figs. 5-6 and 5-7).

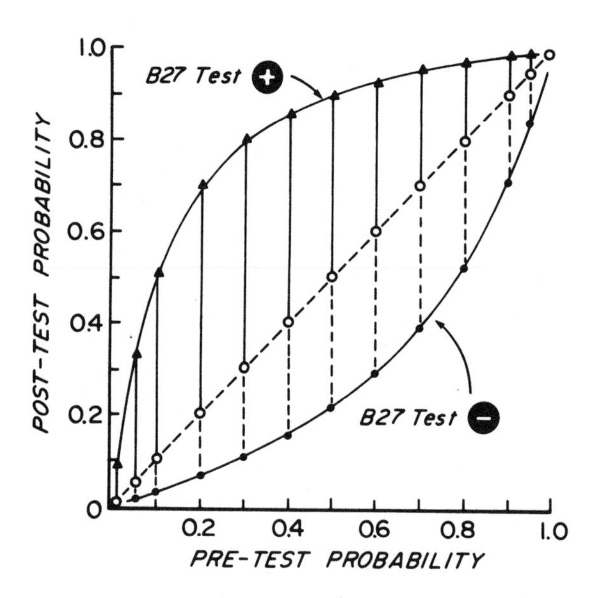

Fig. 5-6. Probability graph describing the predictive value of HLA-B27 testing in Reiter's syndrome in whites. The horizontal axis depicts the physician's estimate of the probability that a patient has the disease before the test is done (pre-test probability). The post-test probability is shown along the vertical axis. The vertical lines indicate the predictive values of the test at different assumed pre-test probabilities. The solid curved lines connect points that indicate post-test probability of disease, following positive (+) or negative (−) B27 test results. (From Khan MA, Khan MK: Diagnostic value of HLA-B27 testing in ankylosing spondylitis or Reiter's syndrome. Ann Intern Med 84:1–7, 1976. With permission.)

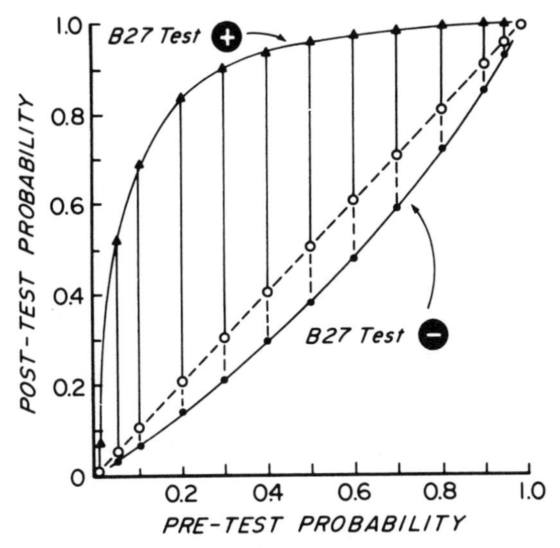

B27 TEST FOR REITER'S SYNDROME IN BLACKS

SENSITIVITY = 40 %
SPECIFICITY = 98 %

Fig. 5-7. Probability graph describing the predictive value of HLA-B27 testing in Reiter's syndrome in blacks. The horizontal axis depicts the physician's estimate of the probability that a patient has the disease before the test is done (pre-test probability). The post-test probability is shown along the vertical axis. The vertical lines indicate the predictive values of the test at different assumed pre-test probabilities. The solid curved lines connect points that indicate post-test probability of disease, following positive (+) or negative (−) B27 test results. (From Khan MA, Khan MK: Diagnostic value of HLA-B27 testing in ankylosing spondylitis or Reiter's syndrome. Ann Intern Med 84:1–7, 1976. With permission.)

SUMMARY

Even early in the course of disease, the diagnosis of AS can usually be made with certainty from history, physical examination, and pelvic x-ray findings alone. In those children and adults whose history and physical examination suggest AS but whose x-ray findings do not permit this diagnosis to be made, the HLA-B27 test may allow the presumptive diagnosis of AS to be accepted or rejected with reasonable certainty. In patients with back pain in whom AS is suggested by neither history nor physical examination,

B27 testing is inappropriate; a positive result would still not permit the diagnosis of AS to be made.

There are a number of reasons to arrive at a correct diagnosis early in the course of AS, even though we do not as yet have a specific treatment. The elimination of uncertainty provides peace of mind for the patient (as well as for the physician), particularly in view of the good prognosis for life and high workplace productivity of AS patients. The patient is spared the fear and insecurity caused by unexplained and undiagnosed back pain, and the occasional imputation of a psychoneurotic basis for the pain is avoided. In addition, unnecessary and potentially harmful diagnostic and therapeutic maneuvers are avoided. Appropriate physical therapy may be undertaken, and the probabilities of a good functional outcome are improved. While the use of phenylbutazone might tend to be avoided in other diseases, establishment of the diagnosis of AS provides justification for the use of this drug in the minds of many rheumatologists; many regard it as the most effective agent in AS.[145,146] As the pathogenesis of AS is elucidated, we can legitimately hope that even better forms of therapy will become available, which make early diagnosis even more important.

REFERENCES

1. Brewerton DA, Hart FD, Nicholls A, et al.: Ankylosing spondylitis and HL-A 27. Lancet 1:904–907, 1973
2. Schlosstein L, Teraski PI, Bluestone R, et al.: High association of an HL-A antigen, W27, with ankylosing spondylitis. N Engl J Med 288:704–706, 1973
3. Wright V: Seronegative polyarthritis: A unified concept. Arthritis Rheum 21:619–633, 1978
4. Moll JMH: Diagnostic criteria and their evaluation, in Moll JMH (ed): Ankylosing Spondylitis. Edinburgh, Churchill Livingstone, 1980
5. Calin A, Fries JF: Striking prevalence of ankylosing spondylitis in "healthy" W27 positive males and females: A controlled study. N Engl J Med 293:835–839, 1975
6. Cohen LM, Mittal KK, Schmid FR, et al.: Increased risk for spondylitis stigmata in apparently healthy HL-AW27 men. Ann Intern Med 84:1–7, 1976
7. Khan MA, Khan MK: Diagnostic value of HLA-B27 testing in ankylosing spondylitis or Reiter's syndrome. Ann Intern Med 96:70–76, 1982

7a. Khan MA: Ankylosing spondylitis, in Calin A (ed): Spondylarthropathies. New York, Grune & Stratton, 1983

8. Moll JMH, Haslock I, Macrae IF, et al.: Association between ankylosing spondylitis, psoriatic arthritis, Reiter's disease, the intestinal arthropathies and Behcet's syndrome. Medicine (Baltimore) 53:343–364, 1974
9. Woodrow JC: Histocompatibility antigens and rheumatic diseases. Semin Arthritis Rheum 6:257–276, 1977
10. Brewerton DA: HLA-B27 and the inheritance of susceptibility to rheumatic disease. Arthritis Rheum 19:656–668, 1976
11. Hochberg MC, Borenstein DG, Arnett FC: The absence of back pain in classical ankylosing spondylitis. John Hopkins Med J 143:181–183, 1978
12. Good AE: Chest pain of ankylosing spondylitis: Its place in the differential diagnosis of heart pain. Ann Intern Med 58:926–937, 1963
13. Hart FD, Bogdanovitch A, Nichol WD: The thorax in ankylosing spondylitis. Ann Rheum Dis 9:116–131, 1950

14. Ogryzlo MA: Ankylosing spondylitis, in Hollander JL, McCarty DJ Jr, (eds): Arthritis and Allied Conditions: A Textbook of Rheumatology, 8th ed. Philadelphia, Lea and Febigor, 1972
15. Riley MJ, Ansell BM, Bywaters EG: Radiological manifestations of ankylosing spondylitis according to age at onset. Ann Rheum Dis 30:138–148, 1971
16. Schaller J. Bitnum S, Wedgewood RJ: Ankylosing spondylitis with childhood onset. J Pediat 74:505–516, 1969
17. Dwosh IL, Resnick D, Becker MA: Hip involvement in ankylosing spondylitis. Arthritis Rheum 19:683–692, 1976.
18. Hart FD, Maclagan NF: Ankylosing spondylitis: A review of 184 cases. Ann Rheum Dis 14:77–83, 1955
19. Davidson C, Wojtulewski JA, Bacon PA, et al.: Temporo-mandibular joint disease in ankylosing spondylitis. Ann Rheum Dis 34:87–91, 1975
20. Rudge SR, Swannell AJ, Rose DH, et al.: The clinical assessment of sacroiliac joint involvement in ankylosing spondylitis. Rheumatol Rehabil 21:15–20, 1981
21. Kellgren JH: Diagnostic criteria for population studies. Bull Rheum Dis 13:291–292, 1962
22. Bennett PH, Wood PHN: Population studies of the rheumatic diseases, in Proceedings of the 3rd International Symposium, New York. Amsterdam, Excerpta Medica Foundation, 1968 (International Congress Series No. 148)
23. Ansell BM: Juvenile spondylitis and related disorders, in Moll JMH, (ed): Ankylosing Spondylitis. Edinburgh, Churchill Livingstone, 1980
24. Thompson GH, Khan MA, Bilenker RM: Spontaneous atlantoaxial subluxation as a presenting manifestation of juvenile ankylosing spondylitis: A case report. Spine 7:78–79, 1982
25. Rosenberg AM, Petty RE: A syndrome of seronegative enthesopathy and arthropathy in children. Arthritis Rheum 25:1041–1047, 1982.
26. Hill HF, Hill AG, Bodmer JG: Clinical diagnosis of ankylosing spondylitis in women and relation to presence of HLA-B27. Ann Rheum Dis 35:267–270, 1976
27. Braunstein EM, Martel W, Moidel R: Ankylosing spondylitis in men and women: A clinical and radiographic comparison. Radiology 144:91–94, 1982
28. Pastershank SP: Ankylosing spondylitis in women. J Can Assoc Radiol 32:93–94, 1981
29. Cheatum DE: HL-A B27 disease in women. Arthritis Rheum 20:761–762, 1977
29a. van der Linden, SM, Valkenburg HA, de Jong BM, et al.: The risk of developing ankylosing spondylitis in HLA-B27 positive individuals: A comparison of relatives of AS patients with the general population. Arthritis Rheum (in press)
30. van der Linden S: Spondylitis ankylopoetica: Een Familie en bevolkingsonderzoek en toetsing van diagnostische criteria (thesis). Leiden, the Netherlands, 1982
31. Resnick D, Dwosh IL, Goergen TG, et al.: Clinical and radiographic abnormalities in ankylosing spondylitis: A comparison of men and women. Diagnost Radiol 119:293–297, 1976
32. Tyson TL, Thompson WAL, Ragan C: Marie-Strumpell spondylitis in women. Ann Rheum Dis 12:40–42, 1953
33. Hart FD, Robinson KC: Ankylosing spondylitis in women. Ann Rheum Dis 18:15–34, 1959
34. McBryde AM Jr, McCollum DE: Ankylosing spondylitis in women: The disease and its prognosis. N Carolina Med J 34:34–37, 1973
35. Goodman CE, Lange RK, Waxman J, et al.: Ankylosing spondylitis in women. Arch Phys Med Rehabil 61:167–170, 1980
36. Carter ET, McKenna, CH, Brian DD, et al.: Epidemiology of ankylosing spondylitis in Rochester, Minnesota, 1935–1973. Arthritis Rheum 22:365–370, 1979
37. Hammoudeh M, Khan MA: Genetics of HLA associated diseases: Ankylosing spondylitis. J Rheumatol 10:301–304, 1983
37a. Khan MA, van der Linden S, Kushner I: Symptomatic ankylosing spondylitis without radiographic sacroiliitis in B27-positive relatives. Clin Res 31:804A, 1983
38. Kozin F, Carrera GF, Ryan LM, et al.: Computed tomography in the diagnosis

of sacroiliitis. Arthritis Rheum 24:1479–1485, 1981
39. Khan MA, Miron SD, Kushner I, et al.: The comparitive value of standard radiography, quantitative scintigraphy and computerized tomography in sacroiliitis. Arthritis Rheum 24 (Suppl):S119, 1981
39a. Miron SD, Khan MA, Wiesen EJ, et al.: The value of quantitative scintigraphy in detection of sacroiliitis. Clin Rheumatol (in press)
40. Carrera GF, Foley WD, Kozin F, et al.: CT of sacroiliitis. AJR 136:41–46, 1981
41. Davis P: Quantitative sacroiliac scintigraphy in ankylosing spondylitis and Crohn's disease: A single family study. Ann Rheum Dis 38:241–243, 1979
42. Esdaile JM, Rosenthall L, Terkeltaub R, et al.: Prospective evaluation of sacroiliac scintigraphy in chronic inflammatory back pain. Arthritis Rheum 23:998–1003, 1980
43. Christiansen FT, Hawkins BR, Dawkins RL, et al.: The prevalence of ankylosing spondylitis among B27 positive normal individuals: A reassessment. J Rheumatol 6:713–718, 1979
44. Dawkins RL, Owen ET, Cheah PS, et al.: Prevalence of ankylosing spondylitis and radiological abnormalities of the sacroiliac joints in HLA-B27 positive individuals (letter). J Rheumatol 8:1025–1026, 1981
45. Boland EW, Present AJ: Rheumatoid spondylitis: A study of one hundred cases, with special reference to diagnostic criteria. JAMA 129:843–849, 1945
46. Moll JMH, Wright V: New York clinical criteria for ankylosing spondylitis: A statistical evaluation. Ann Rheum Dis 32:354–363, 1973
47. Moll JMH, Wright V: The pattern of chest and spinal mobility in ankylosing spondylitis: An objective clinical study of 106 patients. Rheumatol Rehabil 12:115–134, 1973
48. Dihlmann W: Current radiodiagnostic concepts of ankylosing spondylitis. Skeletal Radiol 4:179–188, 1979
49. de Blecourt JJ: 553 patients with ankylosing spondylitis, seen and followed in the period 1948 to 1971. Ann Rheum Dis 32:383–385, 1973
50. Goldin RH, Bluestone R: Tissue typing in rheumatic disease. Clin Rheum Dis 2:231–252, 1976
50a. van der Linden S, Valkenburg HA, Cats A: Evaluation of diagnostic criteria for ankylosing spondylitis: A proposal for modification of The New York criteria. Arthritis Rheum (in press)
50b. van der Linden S, Valkenburg HA, Cats A, et al.: Evaluation of the diagnostic criteria for ankylosing spondylitis: A proposal for modification of The New York criteria. Clin Res 31:734A, 1983
51. Arnett FC Jr, Hochberg MC, Bias WB: Cross-reactive HLA antigens in B27-negative Reiter's syndrome and sacroiliitis. John Hopkins Med J 141:193–197, 1977
52. Daneo V, Migone N, Modena V, et al.: Family studies and HLA typing in ankylosing spondylitis and sacroiliitis. J Rheumatol (Suppl 3) 4:5–10, 1977
53. Möller E, Olhagen B: Studies on the major histocompatibility system in patients with ankylosing spondylitis. Tissue Antigens 6:237–246, 1975
54. Safwenberg J, Doomeij-Nyberg B, Kjallman M: HLA antigens in females with ankylosing spondylitis and other forms of seronegative rheumatic diseases. Scand J Rheumatol 7:177–182, 1978
55. Cowling P, Ebringer R, Ebringer A: Association of inflammation with raised serum IgA in ankylosing spondylitis. Ann Rheum Dis 39:545–549, 1980
56. Kendall MJ, Lawrence DS, Shuttleworth DR, et al.: Hematology and biochemistry of ankylosing spondylitis. Br Med J 2:235–237, 1973
57. Dixon JS, Bird HA, Wright V: A comparison of serum biochemistry in ankylosing spondylitis, seronegative and seropositive rheumatoid arthritis. Ann Rheum Dis 40:404–408, 1981
58. Cowling P, Ebringer R, Ebringer A: Association of inflammation with raised serum IgA in ankylosing spondylitis. Ann Rheum Dis 39:545–549, 1980
59. Bluestone R: Ankylosing spondylitis, in McCarty DJ (ed): Arthritis and Allied Conditions, 9th ed. Philadelphia, Lea and Febiger, 1979

60. Dixon AStJ, Macleod M: Diagnostic problems and differential diagnosis, in Moll JMH (ed): Ankylosing spondylitis. Edinburgh, Churchill Livingstone, 1980
61. Morley J, Kushner I: Serum C-reactive protein levels in disease. Ann NY Acad Sci 389:406–418, 1982
62. Boland EW, Headley NE, Hench PS: The cerebrospinal fluid in rheumatoid spondylitis. Ann Rheum Dis 7:195–199, 1948
63. Kendall MJ, Farr M, Meynell MJ, et al.: Synovial fluid in ankylosing spondylitis. Ann Rheum Dis 32:487–492, 1973
64. Kinsella TD, Espinoza L, Vasey FB: Serum complement and immunoglobulin levels in sporadic and familial ankylosing spondylitis. J Rheumatol 2:308–313, 1975
65. Vinje O, Dobloug JH, Forre O, et al.: Immunoregulatory T cells in the peripheral blood of patients with Bechterew's syndrome. Ann Rheum Dis 41:41–46, 1982
66. Brinch L, Vinje O, Teisberg P, et al.: The in vivo metabolism of C3 in ankylosing spondylitis. Ann Rheum Dis 41:86–89, 1982
67. Maksymowych W, Dasgupta MK, Rothwell RS, et al.: The absence of circulating immune complexes in patients with ankylosing spondylitis. Rheumatol Int 1:107–109, 1981
68. Corrigal V, Panayi GS, Unger A, et al.: Detection of immune complexes in serum of patients with ankylosing spondylitis. Ann Rheum Dis 37:159–163, 1978
69. Holborow EJ, Thompson BR, Howles AD: Biological properties of circulating immune complexes in rheumatoid arthritis, in Panayi GS, Johnson PM (eds): Immunopathogenesis of Rheumatoid Arthritis. Proceedings of the International Symposium held at Guy's Hospital, London, November 1978. Chertsey, England, Reedbooks, 1979
70. Duquesnoy B, Santoro F, Wattre P, et al.: Failure to find Clq-binding material and anti-IgG antibodies in ankylosing spondylitis. Ann Rheum Dis 39:449–452, 1980
71. Greenway GD, Resnick D: Problems in radiographic technique and in radiological assessment of the sacroiliac joints, in Moll JMH (ed): Ankylosing Spondylitis. Edinburgh, Churchill Livingstone, 1980
72. Ball J: Enthesopathy of rheumatoid arthritis and ankylosing spondylitis. Ann Rheum Dis 30:213–223, 1971
73. Cruickshank B: Pathology of ankylosing spondylitis. Clin Orthop 74:43–58, 1971
74. Martel W: Radiological differential diagnosis of ankylosing spondylitis (Bechterew's syndrome). Scand J Rheumatol (Suppl 32):141–156, 1980
75. McEwen C, DiTata D, Lingg C, et al.: Ankylosing spondylitis and spondylitis accompanying ulcerative colitis, regional enteritis, psoriasis and Reiter's disease: A comparative study. Arthritis Rheum 14:291–318, 1971
76. Bowen V, Cassidy JD: Macroscopic and microscopic anatomy of the sacroiliac joint from embryonic life until the eighth decade. Spine 6:620–628, 1981
77. Cohen AS, McNeil JM, Calkins E, et al.: The normal sacroiliac joint: Analysis of 88 sacroiliac roentgenograms. AJR 100:559–563, 1967
78. Resnick D, Niwayama G: Ankylosing spondylitis, in Resnick D, Niwayama G (eds): Diagnosis of Bone and Joint Disorders. Philadelphia, W.B. Saunders, 1981
79. Forestier J, Lagier R: Ankylosing hyperostosis of the spine. Clin Orthop 74:65–83, 1971
79a. Yagan R, Khan MA: Confusion of roentgenographic differential diagnosis between ankylosing hyperostosis (Forestier's disease) and ankylosing spondylitis. Clin Rheumatol 2:285–292, 1983
80. Shapiro RF, Wiesner KB, Bryan BL, et al.: HLA-B27 and modified bone formation. Lancet 1:230–231, 1976
81. Rosenthal M, Bahous I, Muller W: Increased frequency of HLA-B8 in hyperostotic spondylosis. J Rheumatol 4 (Suppl 3):94–96, 1977
82. Brigode M, Francois RJ: Histocompatibility antigens in vertebral ankylosing hyperostosis. J Rheumatol 4:429–434, 1977
83. Jumshyd A, Khan MA: Ankylosing hyperostosis in American Blacks: A

prospective study. Clin Rheumatol 2:123–126, 1983
84. Franck WA, Bress NM, Singer FR, et al.: Rheumatic manifestations of Paget's disease of bone. Am J Med 56:592–603, 1974
85. Singh A, Dass R, Hayreh SS, et al.: Skeletal changes in endemic fluorosis. J Bone Joint Surg [Br] 44B:806–815, 1962
86. Brem JB: Vertebral ankylosis in a patient with hereditary chondrocalcinosis: A chance association? Arthritis Rheum 25:1257–1263, 1982
87. Reginato AJ, Schiapachasse V, Zmijewski CM, et al.: HLA antigens in chondrocalcinosis and ankylosing chondrocalcinosis. Arthritis Rheum 22:928–932, 1979
88. Jimenea CV, Frame B, Chaykin LB, et al.: Spondylitis of hypoparathyroidism. Clin Orthop 74:84–89, 1971
89. Bywaters EGL, Dixon ASJ, Scott ST: Joint lesions of hyperparathyroidism. Ann Rheum Dis 22:171–187, 1963
90. Resnick D, Dwosh IL, Niwayama G: Sacroiliac joint in renal osteodystrophy: Roentgenographic-pathologic correlation. J Rheumatol 2:287–295, 1975
91. Khan MA, Kushner I, Freehafer AA: Sacroiliac joint abnormalities in paraplegics. Ann Rheum Dis 38:317–319, 1979
92. Bhate DV, Pizarro AJ, Seitam A, et al.: Axial skeletal changes in paraplegics. Radiology 133:55–58, 1979
93. Hunter T, Hildahl CR, Smith NJ, et al.: Histocompatibility antigens in paraplegic or quadriplegic patients with sacroiliac joint changes. J Rheumatol 6:92–95, 1979
94. De Bosset P, Gordon DA, Smythe HA, et al.: Comparison of osteitis condensans ilii and ankylosing spondylitis in female patients: Clinical, radiological and HLA typing characteristics. J Chron Dis 31:171–181, 1978
95. Calin A: Ankylosing spondylitis sine sacroiliitis. Arthritis Rheum 22:303–304, 1979
96. Lambert JR, Wright V: Psoriatic spondylitis: A clinical and radiological description of the spine in psoriatic arthritis. Q J Med 46:411–425, 1977
97. Hounsfield GN: Computerized transverse, axial scanning (tomography). Br J Radiol 46:1016–1012, 1973
98. Relman AS: CAT scanners—conferring "the greatest benefit on mankind" (editorial). N Engl J Med 301:1062–1063, 1979
99. Borlaza GS, Seigel R, Kuhns LR, et al.: Computed tomography in the evaluation of sacroiliac arthritis. Radiology 139:437–440, 1981
100. Kramer LD, Krouth GJ: Computerized tomography: An adjunct to early diagnosis in the cauda equina syndrome of ankylosing spondylitis. Arch Neurol 35:116–118, 1978
101. Ullrich CG, Binet EF, Sinecki MG, et al.: Quantitative assessment of lumbar spinal canal by computed tomography. Radiology 134: 137–143, 1980
102. Haughton VM, Syverstsen A, William AL: Soft tissue anatomy within the spinal canal as seen on computed tomography. Radiology 134:649–655, 1980
103. Genant HK, Cann CE, Chafetz NI, et al.: Advances in computed tomography of the musculoskeletal system. Radiol Clin North Am 19:645–674, 1981
104. Williams AL, Haughton VM, Syvertsen A: Computed tomography in the diagnosis of herniated nucleus pulposus. Radiology 135:95–99, 1980
105. Cacayorin ED, Kieffer SA: Applications and limitations of computed tomography of the spine. Radiol Clin North Am 20:185–206, 1982
106. Handel SF, Lee Y: Computed tomography of spinal fractures. Radiol Clin North Am 19:69–89, 1981
107. Seltzer SE, Weissman BN, Finberg HF, et al.: Improved diagnostic imaging in joint disease. Semin Arthritis Rheum 11:315–330, 1982
108. Greyson ND: Radionuclide bone and joint imaging in rheumatology. Bull Rheum Dis 30:1034–1039, 1979
109. Ho G Jr, Sadovnikoff N, Malhotra CM, et al.: Quantitative sacroiliac joint scintigraphy: A critical assessment. Arthritis Rheum 22:837–844, 1979
110. Rothwell RS, Davis P, Lentle BC: Radionuclide bone scanning in females

with chronic low back pain. Ann Rheum Dis 40:79–82, 1981
111. Domeij-Nyberg B, Kjällman M, Pettersson N-O: The reliability of quantitative bone scanning in sacro-iliitis. Scand J Rheumatol 9:77–79, 1980
112. Namey TC, McIntyre J, Buse M, et al.: Nucleographic studies of axial spondarthritis. I. Quantitative sacroiliac scintigraphy in early HLA-B27-associated sacroiliitis. Arthritis Rheum 20:1058–1064, 1977
113. Szanto, E: Quantitative sacro-iliac 99m TC-pertechnetate scanning (QTPS): an analysis of the clinical usefulness for the detection of inflammation of the sacroiliac joints. Scand J Rheumatol (Suppl 32): 130–132, 1980
114. Dequeker J, Goddeeris T, Walravens M, et al.: Evaluation of sacroiliitis: comparison of radiological and radionuclide techniques. Radiology 128:687–689, 1978
115. Green FA: Joint scintiscans: present status (Editorial). J Rheumatol 6:370–373, 1979
116. Munkner T: Scintigraphic methods and possibilities. Scand J Rheumatol (Suppl 32):120–123, 1980
117. Spencer DG, Adams FG, Horton PW, et al.: Scintiscanning in ankylosing spondylitis: A clinical, radiological and quantitative radioisotopic study. J Rheumatol 6:426, 1979
118. Gelman MI, Coleman RE, Stevens PM, et al.: Radiography, radionuclide imaging, and arthrography in the evaluation of total hip and knee replacement. Radiology 128:677–682, 1978
119. Williamson BR, McLaughlin RE, Wang G-J, et al.: Radionuclide bone imaging as a means of differentiating loosening and infection in patients with a painful hip prosthesis. Radiology 133:723–725, 1979
120. Grennan DM, Caygill L: Infra-red thermography in the assessment of sacroiliac inflammation. Rheumatol Rehabil 21:81–87, 1982
121. McCullough EC, Baker HL Jr: Nuclear magnetic resonance imaging. Radiol Clin North Am 20:3–7, 1982
122. Khan MA: Clinical application of the HLA-B27 test in rheumatic disease: A current perspective. Arch Inter Med 140:177–180, 1980
123. Hawkins BR, Dawkins RL, Christiansen FT, et al.: Use of the B27 test in the diagnosis of ankylosing spondylitis: A statistical evaluation. Arthritis Rheum 24:743–746, 1981
124. Calin A: HLA-B27: To type or not to type?: Ann Intern Med 92 (Part I):208–211, 1980
125. Golding DN, Jenkins WJ: Histocompatibility testing in doubtful cases of ankylosing spondylitis. Lancet 2:522–523, 1974
126. Joysey VC, Wolf E: HLA-A, -B and -C antigens, their serology and cross reaction. Br Med Bull 34:217–222, 1978
127. Grumet FC, Fendly BM, Engleman EG: Monoclonal anti-HLA-B27 antibody (B27M1): Production and lack of detectable typing difference between patients with ankylosing spondylitis, Reiter's syndrome and normal controls. Lancet 2:174–176, 1981
128. Ellis SA, Taylor C, McMichael A: Recognition of HLA-B27 and related antigen by a monoclonal antibody. Hum Immunol 5:49–59, 1982
129. Grumet FC, Fendly BM, Fish L, et al.: Monoclonal antibody (B27M2) subdividing HLA-B27. Hum Immunol 5:61–72, 1982
130. Khan MA, Kushner I, Braun WE: Comparison of clinical features in HLA-B27 positive and negative patients with ankylosing spondylitis. Arthritis Rheum 20:909–912, 1977
131. Khan MA, Braun WE, Kushner I, et al.: HLA-B27 in ankylosing spondylitis: Differences in frequency and relative risk in American Blacks and Caucasians. J Rheumatol 4 (Suppl 3):39–43, 1977
132. Khan MA, Kushner I, Braun WE: Genetic heterogeneity in primary ankylosing spondylitis. J Rheumatol 7:383–386, 1980
133. Khan MA, Askari AD, Braun WE, et al.: Low association of HLA-B27 with Reiter's syndrome in blacks. Ann Intern Med 90:202–203, 1979
134. Arnett FC, McClusky OE, Schacter BZ, et al.: Incomplete Reiter's syndrome:

Discriminating features and HLA-W27 in diagnosis. Ann Intern Med 84:8–12, 1976

135. Arnett FC: Incomplete Reiter's syndrome: Clinical comparisons with classical triad. Ann Rheum Dis 38 (Suppl 1):73–78, 1979
136. McCord WC, Nies KM, Louie JS: Acute venereal arthritis: Comparative study of acute Reiter's syndrome and acute gonococcal arthritis. Arch Intern Med 137:858–862, 1977
137. Morris R, Metzger AL, Bluestone R, et al.: HL-A W27: A clue to the diagnosis and pathogenesis of Reiter's syndrome. N Engl J Med 290:554–556, 1974
138. Aho K, Ahvonen P, Lassus A, et al.: HL-A 27 in reactive arthritis: A study of Yersinis arthritis and Reiter's disease. Arthritis Rheum 17:521–526, 1974
139. Hakansson U, Low B, Eitrem R, et al.: HL-A 27 and reactive arthritis in an outbreak of salmonellosis. Tissue Antigens 6;366–367, 1975
140. Leirisalo M, Skylv G, Kousa M, et al.: Followup study on patients with Reiter's disease and reactive arthritis, with special reference to HLA-B27. Arthritis Rheum 25:249–259, 1982
141. Griner PF, Mayewski RJ, Mushlin AL, et al.: Selection and interpretation of diagnostic tests and procedures: Principles and applications. Ann Intern Med 94 (Part 2):553–600, 1981
142. Bryant GD, Norman GR: Expressions of probability: Words and numbers. N Engl J Med 302:411, 1980
143. Eddy DM, Clanton CH: The art of diagnosis: Solving the clinicopathological exercise. N Engl J Med 306:1263–1268, 1982
144. Boersma JW: Retardation of ossification of the lumbar vertebral column in ankylosing spondylitis by means of phenylbutazone. Scand J Rheumatol 5:60–64, 1976
145. Calabro JJ: An appraisal of the medical and surgical management of ankylosing spondylitis. Clin Orthop 60:125–148, 1968
146. Calin A, Marks S: Management of ankylosing spondylitis. Bull Rheum Dis 31:35–38, 1981

Don L. Goldenberg
Peter A. Rice

6

Disseminated Gonococcal Infection: Current Understanding of the Clinical Manifestations, Laboratory Features, and Pathogenesis

CLINICAL MANIFESTATIONS OF DISSEMINATED GONOCOCCAL INFECTION

Initial Symptoms

Most patients with disseminated gonococcal infection (DGI) experience migratory or additive polyarthralgias as early symptoms (Table 6-1). These symptoms may involve only a single joint, are usually transient, and may be associated with objective signs of synovitis or tenosynovitis. Constitutional features such as fever, chills, and headache are common. Twenty-five percent of our patients initially noted skin lesions, but only 17 percent initially complained of local genitourinary symptoms. Dermatitis and urethritis are often asymptomatic throughout the course of DGI. Although most patients seek medical attention within 2–4 days of the onset of symptoms, some will be symptomatic for 1 week or longer prior to hospitalization; and the median duration of symptoms prior to hospitalization in our experience was 4 days.[1]

Demographic Features

In the preantibiotic era, DGI was much more common in males. In the past 20 years, however, female predominance has emerged. In our recent experience, (the past 7 years), there were 35 women and 13 men with DGI.

PROGRESS IN CLINICAL RHEUMATOLOGY VOL. I ISBN 0-8089-1646-7

Table 6-1
Initial Symptoms of DGI*

Symptoms	(%)
Polyarthralgias	65
Monarthralgia	25
Dermatitis	25
Fever, chills	31
Genitourinary symptoms	17

*Symptoms derived from patients' history in our recent experience, 1975–1981.
From O'Brien JP, Goldenberg DL, Rice PA: Disseminated gonococcal infection: A clinical and laboratory survey of 49 patients. Medicine, 62:395–406, 1983. With permission.

The patients are usually between the ages of 15 and 35, although DGI has been reported in the very young[2,3] and the very old.[4] Often a history of recent sexual contact is denied. Our patients have reported that their last sexual contact was anywhere from 1 day to 2 months prior to the onset of symptoms of DGI. Therefore, the usual duration of an asymptomatic stage of DGI is not known.

Recurrent episodes of DGI are not common and usually occur in patients with complement–component deficiencies.[5,6] Twenty-five percent of our patients, however, admitted to prior episodes of gonorrhea. The initial manifestations of DGI are often temporally related to menstruation or pregnancy in females.[7,8] Thus, most women note the onset of DGI within one week of their last menstrual period. It has been postulated that cervical pH changes and microbial virulence factors select more virulent strains of DGI during menstruation.[1] Some reports describe an increased frequency of DGI in homosexuals and intravenous drug users.[1]

Physical Examination

The musculoskeletal manifestations of DGI are the prominent feature. Whereas a single, hot, swollen joint is characteristic of nongonococcal bacterial, arthritis, tenosynovitis, and polyarthritis are more typical of DGI (Table 6-2). For example, in a recent report, tenosynovitis was present in 68 percent of patients, polyarthritis in 52 percent, and monarthritis in 48 percent.[9] In our series, 67 percent had tenosynovitis, 67 percent had dermatitis, 63 percent had fever, 42 percent had arthritis, and 25 percent had genitourinary symptoms at the time of initial physical examination (Table 6-3). The variable descriptions of these musculoskeletal manifestations may be related to the authors' definition of arthritis and tenosynovitis. For example, our criterion for arthritis required the demonstration of purulent synovial

Table 6-2
Differential Features of Gonococcal and Nongonococcal Bacterial Arthritis

Gonococcal Arthritis	Nongonococcal Bacterial Arthritis
Usually healthy, young adults	Often compromised host, often very young or aged
Tenosynovitis often	No tenosynovitis
Polyarthritis common	Monarthritis common
Skin lesions in two-thirds	No associated dermatitis
Wrists and small joints common	Large joints predominate
Migratory polyarthralgias	No prodromal joint symptoms
Synovial fluid culture positive in less than 50%	Synovial fluid cultures are usually positive
Blood cultures rarely positive	Blood cultures positive in 50% of patients
Rapid and complete response to antibiotics	Slower response to antibiotics (joint drainage important)

fluid with greater than 25,000 leukocytes/mm^3. In recent reports, tenosynovitis has been more common than arthritis and has been present in 66 percent of patients with DGI.[1] It is not clear whether the increased frequency of tenosynovitis is related to a true change in the clinical manifestations or is due to a greater appreciation and definition of tenosynovitis (rather than including all joint symptoms as arthritis). The tenosynovitis usually involved multiple joints, especially the wrists, fingers, toes, and ankles.

Monarthritis or polyarthritis has been present in less than 50 percent of patients in recent series of DGI.[1,9] Twenty of 48 (42 percent) of our DGI patients had purulent arthritis defined by synovial fluid analysis. The knee has been the most commonly affected joint, which may, in part, reflect the ease of diagnosis and aspiration of a knee joint effusion. The synovial fluid

Table 6-3
Presenting Features at the Time of Initial Hospitalization of 48 Patients with DGI*

Feature	No. of Patients (%)
Tenosynovitis	32 (67)
Dermatitis	32 (67)
Fever	30 (63)
Arthritis	20 (42)
Genitourinary symptoms	12 (25)

From O'Brien JP, Goldenberg DL, Rice PA: Disseminated gonococcal infection: A clinical and laboratory survey of 49 patients. Medicine 62:395–406, 1983. With permission.

leukocyte count has ranged between 40,000 and 60,000 cells/mm^3 in most series. The percentage of polymorphonuclear leukocytes has been over 80 percent, and there is often a depression of the synovial fluid glucose in relationship to the blood glucose. The mean synovial fluid leukocyte counts, however, have not been quite as elevated as those described in staphylococcal and other types of nongonococcal bacterial arthritis.[10] All joints, including the hip and shoulder, have been affected. The sacroiliac joint, temporomandibular, and sternoclavicular joints are rarely involved.[11,12]

The other most common abnormality on physical examination is dermatitis, which has been present in about 66 percent of patients. The skin lesions are usually multiple and are found most commonly on the arms and legs, sometimes on the trunk, but rarely on the face, hands, or feet. They are usually painless and patients are often unaware of their presence. Occasionally they may be painful and may even appear pustular or resemble vasculitis. Most common are small macules or papules. Any form of skin lesion has been associated with DGI, however; this includes pustules, vesicles, bullae, erythema nodosum, or erythema multiforme. Sometimes new skin lesions will develop despite the initiation of appropriate antibiotic therapy. As discussed below, the skin lesions are almost always sterile. Although most patients with DGI are febrile and often describe shaking chills, almost 40 percent of patients do not have any substantial fever once hospitalized. The mean temperature of our patients was 100.0°F, and the mean peripheral blood leukocyte count was 11,000 cells/mm^3. Most patients deny any local genitourinary, rectal, or throat symptoms, despite the fact that *Neisseria gonorrhoeae* is often recovered from these local sites. In the postantibiotic era, gonococcal meningitis and endocarditis have been rarely reported.[1,13] There have been a few reports of a presumed immune-mediated glomerulonephritis secondary to DGI.[14]

Four of our patients had transiently elevated hepatocellular enzymes without an obvious etiology other than DGI. It is not clear whether this is a result of a transient septicemia or related to the Fitz–Hugh–Curtis syndrome, a perihepatitis,[15] which occurs in women and is due to adhesions between the parietal surface of the liver and the peritoneum; it is a result of hematogenous seeding or direct intraperitoneal spread of the organisms. In this situation abdominal pain, tenderness, and signs of pelvic inflammatory disease develop; the diagnosis can be confirmed by laparoscopy. Our patients with abnormal liver function studies, however, were asymptomatic and the abnormal liver function studies quickly normalized with antibiotic treatment.

Results of Culture

The genitourinary tract provides the best opportunity to recover *N. gonorrhoeae* despite the fact that localized genitourinary symptoms are infrequent (Table 6-4). Eighty percent of our patients with DGI had positive

Table 6-4
Isolation of *N. gonorrhoeae* from Various Culture Sites (% Positive)

Author (Ref)	Genitourinary	Pharynx	Rectum	Synovial Fluid	Blood	Skin
Brogadir et al[9]	81	17	13	29	4	0
O'Brien et al[1]	80	10	21	27	5	0

cultures for *N. gonorrhoeae* from a genitourinary site. The organisms can be recovered from the synovial fluid in about 25 percent of the patients and can only rarely be recovered from the blood or from the skin lesions. There have been rare reports of concurrently positive blood and synovial fluid cultures (Table 6-5)[1,7,9,16–19].

Sequential Stages of Disseminated Gonococcal Infection

There has been significant controversy in the literature regarding the concept of sequential clinical stages in DGI. Keiser et al.[16] and Holmes et al.[7] popularized the concept of an initial bacteremic phase that is usually associated with dermatitis and tenosynovitis followed by a joint localization stage (Table 6-6). Other authors reported, however, that there was too much overlap to consider such a temporal sequence of clinical events. For example, 4 of 5 major reviews of DGI since 1974 did not report a significant difference in the duration of symptoms prior to hospitalization for patients with purulent arthritis versus those with dermatitis and tenosynovitis (Table 6-6). Most reports have also concluded that dermatitis is much more common in patients

Table 6-5
The Isolation of *N. gonorrhoeae* from the Blood and/or Synovial Fluid in DGI

Blood Only	Synovial Fluid Only	Both Sites	Author (Ref)
6	9	0	Keiser et al (16)
9	6	2	Holmes et al (7)
7	15	0	Brandt et al (17)
5	20	1	Gelfand et al (18)
7	4	1	Thompson et al (19)
3	10	0	Brogadir et al (9)
13	9	0	O'Brien et al (1)
50	73	4	

Table 6-6
Are There Sequential Clinical Stages in DGI?

Author (ref)	Association of dermatitis and Tenosynovitis (duration prior to hospitalization)	Association of dermatitis and Purulent Arthritis (duration prior to hospitalization)
Keiser et al (16)	5 of 6 (2.7 days)	1 of 9 (5.9 days)
Brandt et al (17)	4 of 7 (2.3 days)	2 of 15 (3.4 days)
Gelfand et al (18)	17 of 17 (3.7 days)	4 of 24 (8 days)
Goldman (20)	5 of 8 (2 days)	2 of 4 (3.2 days)
Brogadir et al (9)	8 of 12 (4.3 days)	11 of 22 (4.9 days)
O'Brien et al (1)	25 of 30 (4 days)	8 of 19 (4 days)

with tenosynovitis (80 percent) than those with purulent arthritis (30 percent) (Table 6-6). Many investigators, therefore, now favor a continuum of DGI during which signs of sepsis may be more prominent earlier in the disease. Clinical subgroups sometimes, but not always, are identifiable.

Our own data support the concept of significant overlap in sequential stages and the presence of clinical subgroups.[1] We believe that an overemphasis on temporal, sequential manifestations may have obscured the relationship that these manifestations have to host and to microbial factors. In examining the relationship of the clinical manifestations to microbial factors in DGI, for example, it was found that *N. gonorrhoeae* strains isolated from patients with purulent arthritis had phenotypic characteristics that differed from those isolated from patients with dermatitis and tenosynovitis.[20]

Treatment of Disseminated Gonococcal Infection

The outlook of patients with DGI is usually one of rapid and complete recovery. With appropriate antibiotic therapy, the fever and clinical symptoms are usually eradicated in a few days.[21–25] Many different antibiotic regimens have been found to be equally effective (Table 6-7). The therapeutic response is so dramatic that it has often served as a diagnostic guide.[7,11] In contrast to patients with nongonococcal bacterial arthritis, patients with DGI usually do not require repeated mechanical joint drainage and almost never require open surgical drainage, even when hips or shoulders are infected.[1]

Occasionally patients will not respond to treatment as rapidly and completely. For example, those with large, purulent joint effusions may require prolonged hospitalization, and their effusions may not clear for days or even for weeks (see page 193, The role of immune or hypersensitivity phenomena). Indeed, the presence of a large, purulent joint effusion is the single most important factor that determines the length of hospitalization in patients with DGI.[23] Recently there have been a few reports of penicillinase-producing

Table 6-7
Antibiotic Regimens Found to Eradicate DGI

Author (ref)	Antibiotic	Dose	Route	Duration
Holmes et al (7)	Penicillin	10 million units	IV, then po	10–14 days
Garcia-Kutzbach et al (21)	Penicillin	1.2–2.4 million units	IV or IM	7–10 days
Blankenship et al (22)	Penicillin	10 million units	IV	3 days
Handsfield et al (23)	Penicillin	10 million	IV	1–5 days
	and ampicillin	2 g	po	7–10 days
	or ampicillin	3.5 g initially,	po	
		then 2 g		7 days
Trentham et al (24)	Penicillin	1.2 million units	IM	10 days
Thompson et al (25)	Erythromycin	2 g	po	7 days

strains of *N. gonorrhoeae*.[26] These strains will obviously not respond quickly or completely to the usual antibiotic regimen and clearly a diagnostic trial of penicillin will not be useful in such a circumstance. Spectinomycin and some of the newer cephalosporins have been effective in treating such resistant strains.

Although not all patients with DGI require hospitalization,[24] we recommend parenteral antibiotic therapy in the hospital. Two or 3 days of hospitalization are usually adequate to assess the response to treatment and allow enough time for all culture results to return. Patients with a purulent joint effusion should be hospitalized, and 7–10 days of therapy may be required with repeated mechanical joint drainage and nonweight bearing. Hospitalization is mandatory when the diagnosis is not certain or when the patient is not reliable. The strains that cause DGI are, in general, more sensitive to penicillin than are strains that cause local genitourinary infection; therefore, massive doses of antibiotics are usually not needed.[27] Since the recovery of *N. gonorrhoeae* from the synovial fluid, from the blood, or from the skin is possible in less than 50 percent of patients, a therapeutic trial of antibiotics that result in a rapid response will often be very helpful for diagnostic purposes.

Differential Diagnosis

DGI should be the leading diagnostic consideration in any sexually active patient who presents with polyarthritis or monarthritis. If tenosynovitis and/or dermatitis are also present, the diagnosis is very likely to be DGI; therefore, antibiotics should be initiated following all appropriate cultures. Any joint effusion should be aspirated and immediately plated on chocolate agar or Thayer—Martin media as well as on plain blood agar. A Gram stained smear of concentrated synovial fluid is useful but will be positive in only approximately 25 percent of DGI joint effusions. The synovial fluid leukocyte count is usually 40,000–60,000 cell/mm^3, although more variability exists than in nongonococcal bacterial effusions. Blood cultures should always be obtained as well as appropriate genitourinary cultures, although the yield is low (see Table 6-4). The genitourinary, anal, and pharyngeal cultures should be plated on selected media such as Thayer–Martin or modified New York City media to inhibit nonneisserial pathogens from overgrowing the culture plate. The endocervical canal provides the highest culture yield in the female. Urethral exudates of both females and males should be obtained; if there is no spontaneous discharge, secretions should be expressed by massaging the urethra in the female or the prostate in the male.

The differential diagnosis of DGI includes hepatitis, Reiter's syndrome, acute rheumatic fever, bacterial endocarditis, other viremias and septicemias, and other connective tissue diseases (Table 6-8). Polyarthritis, as well as tenosynovitis, will occur commonly in the "prodrome" of hepatitis. A skin rash is also common, although the rash is more often urticarial. If synovial effusions can be aspirated, the characteristic leukocyte count is usually less than in gonococcal arthritis, although variable counts have been reported. The major diagnostic clue will be the clinical and laboratory evidence of hepatitis. Positive serologic tests for HBsAg and the absence of positive cultures for *N. gonorrhoeae* will help to confirm the diagnosis.

Reiter's syndrome also commonly presents with an asymmetrical arthritis, tenosynovitis, and urethritis. Some Scandinavian investigators believe that gonococcal urethritis may cause Reiter's syndrome.[28] Nevertheless, most reports describe Reiter's syndrome only in association with nongonococcal urethritis. Helpful differential features include the presence of conjunctivitis and the characteristic mucocutaneous lesions of Reiter's syndrome, such as circinate balanitis and keratodermia blennorrhagica. Clinical or radiologic evidence of sacroilitis and the presence of HLA-B27 will also be supporting evidence for Reiter's syndrome.

Acute rheumatic fever often presents in young adults as a polyarthritis without evidence of carditis, chorea, or subcutaneous nodules. If a skin rash is present, it is usually evanescent and associated with fever. A recent streptococcal throat infection documented clinically or with appropriate culture and serologic tests is necessary for a confirmatory diagnosis. Patients usually respond quite well and rapidly to salicylates.

Bacterial endocarditis as well as other forms of bacteremia can also cause musculoskeletal and dermatologic manifestations that may mimic DGI. Positive blood cultures should establish the diagnosis. Similarly, viremia such as seen in rubella can cause an acute arthritis and a skin rash. Juvenile rheumatoid arthritis, rheumatoid arthritis, systemic lupus erythematosus, and other connective tissue disorders can also begin so explosively that they may suggest DGI. The subsequent clinical course will be necessary for the diagnosis of those more chronic conditions.

Table 6-8
The Differential Diagnosis of DGI

Illness	Polyarthritis	Tenosynovitis	Dermatitis	Sex	Laboratory	Other helpful differential features
DGI	+ +	+ +	+ + (Maculopapular vesicles, pustules)	> Females	Positive culture	Response to antibiotics
Hepatitis	+ +	+ +	+ (Urticaria, macules, papules)	Female-male	Abnormal liver function tests, HB_sAg	Clinical evidence of hepatitis
Reiter's syndrome	+ +	+	+ (Nail lesions, keratodermia)	> Males	HLA B27	Conjunctivitis, sacroiliitis, oral lesions, balanitis
Acute rheumatic fever	+ +	+	Rare	Female-male	Positive throat culture or seriologic evidence of streptococcus B infection	Carditis, response to salicylates

The "diagnostic response" to antibiotics can be helpful in DGI and once all cultures have been obtained, a patient with suspected DGI should be started on antibiotics. As mentioned earlier, however, the blood and synovial fluid are often sterile. Even the genitourinary tract may not yield the organisms and, thus, there will be no positive cultures, and a diagnosis will be a presumptive one. Investigators have referred to such cases as possible DGI, those with positive local cultures as probable DGI, and those with positive blood or synovial fluid cultures as definite or proven cases of DGI. In view of the frequency of negative cultures from the local as well as disseminate sites, however, such classifications provide little therapeutic or clinical utility.

MICROBIAL AND HOST FEATURES OF DISSEMINATED GONOCOCCAL INFECTION

Microbial and Virulence Factors Associated with Disseminated Gonococcal Infection

Neisseria gonorrhoeae are Gram-negative diplococci that can be characterized by their ability of oxidize N-N-dimethyl-*p*-phenylenediamine hydrochloride (positive oxidase test) and by their specific sugar fermentation patterns, which provides differentiation from other *Neisseria* species. Strains that cause disseminated disease are further distinguished by their fastidious growth requirements.[29] Examples of these growth requirements include the pinpoint colonies seen on standard chocolate agar and the frequent inability or delay of the growth or organisms in standard broths used to culture blood. DGI strains are relatively more capneiophilic (CO_2 requiring) than many local strains and are best grown in conditions that provide supplemental CO_2 (4–8 percent), such as a candle extinction jar or a CO_2 incubator.

Strains that cause disseminated disease have been found to possess several unique phenotypic features, such as unique nutritional requirements and enhanced sensitivity to penicillin, that may differentiate them from many strains that cause symptomatic local disease only.[30] We found that 58 percent of DGI strains possessed the nutritional requirement for arginine, hypoanthine and uracil (Arg^-, Hyx^-, Ura^- auxotypes), with or without a proline requirement,[1] a finding similar to that reported for DGI strains from other geographic locales.[30] In contrast, only 8 percent of the strains from cases of uncomplicated gonorrhoeae in Boston are of the Arg^- Hyx^- Ura^- auxotype.[1] The DGI strains in our series also had a mean inhibitory concentration (MIC) to penicillin of 0.0527 ug/ml, whereas the MICs of organisms that cause pelvic inflammatory disease was 0.14 ug/ml. Attempts to link genetic mutations to low level penicillin sensitivity with these organisms' propensity to disseminate have not been successful.[29] None of the strains isolated from the patient with DGI were penicillinase producing, although more examples of penicillinase-producing strains causing DGI have recently been reported.[26]

What characteristics are responsible for these strains' differences? Numerous antigenic structures of gonococci, such as their lipopolysaccharide (LPS)[31] and their pili,[32] contain antigenic determinants that may be responsible for relative and specific types of virulence. The human immune response to these antigens may also be involved in the diverse clinical response to gonococcal strains. The antigenic diversity of gonococci and the specificity of protective human antibodies for gonococcal determinants may explain the apparent lack of protective immunity in much of the local disease caused by *N. gonorrhoeae*. For example, initial bouts of gonococcal pelvic inflammatory disease preclude subsequent bouts caused by the same outer membrane protein serotype,[33] and recurrent DGI is rare unless the host is deficient in complement.[5,6] These observations suggest that invasive gonococcal infection may result in highly specific protective immunity, effective only against subsequent invasive but not mucosal disease. The presence of unique principal outer membrane protein antigens on DGI strains has been demonstrated in our studies by the predominance of the CoA-1 serotype and, more specifically, by other investigators who have demonstrated one or two outer membrane serotypes in most of the strains.[34] These have been characterized on SDS-polyacrylamide gel electrophoresis to be similar-sized principal outer-membrane protein termed protein 1.

Interactions of the Host with *N. gonorrhoeae* that Cause Disseminated Gonococcal Infection

Women are more likely to develop DGI than men, a finding that has been reported in numerous studies.[1,9,17] Menses and pregnancy are risk factors. Ten of our 35 female patients had just completed their menses and 4 others were pregnant at the onset of DGI. Gonococci change their colonial phenotype during menses.[35] This is characterized by a change from the opaque to the transparent colony types, which are more invasive. They are also more resistant to the killing action of normal human serum (NHS) than opaque strains.[35] In our study, the transparent strains were more frequently isolated from disseminated sites of infection.[1] The changes in the endometrium or cervix associated with menses and pregnancy may select more virulent strains and account for the female prevalence of DGI. Pharyngeal colonization may also be important in DGI as a potential site of entry into the bloodstream.

Males with gonorrhoeae are often asymptomatic and the diagnosis is often not evident, whereas local gonococcal infection in women is often associated with a cervical discharge. Furthermore, a significant number of these women develop abdominal pain, adnexal tenderness, or frank pelvic inflammatory disease. In contrast, some patients with DGI report prolonged periods of time from their last sexual exposure to the onset of their initial symptoms. Only 7 of our DGI patients, however, presented with local genitourinary, rectal, or oral symptoms.[1] None of our female patients had symptoms or clinical evidence of pelvic inflammatory disease at the onset of DGI.

Strains that produce asymptomatic local disease in some geographic locales share similar features to DGI strains, such as the mutual possession of the Arg^- Hyx^- Ura^- auxotype[30] and the ability of both to resist the complement dependent bacteriolysis of normal human sera (NHS). These features may be related to the impaired ability of these strains to generate complement-dependent chemotaxis of polymorphonuclear leukocytes in NHS compared to strains that cause pelvic inflammatory disease.[36] Thus, the absence of local symptoms or pelvic inflammatory disease in patients with DGI may be related to the fact that complement activation by DGI strains does not result in enough inflammation at the mucosal site to contain the local infection.

The marked difference in the DGI and local strains to resist or to be killed by normal human serum also may help to determine the clinical manifestations of each strain. Our prospective clinical analysis of DGI patients found that the strains isolated from these patients could be separated into one of two clinical subgroups related to NHS sensitivity. No group I strains were sensitive to each of 19 NHS tested, whereas many group II organisms were more sensitive (Table 6-9). The sensitivity of these group II strains that cause suppurative arthritis more closely resembles that of pelvic inflammatory disease strains, and both may cause significant local inflammation. The escape of a particular strain of *N. gonorrhoeae* from the mucosal site to the bloodstream may, therefore in part, be the result of that particular infected host's failure to mount a local response. The absence of bactericidal activity in early serum samples from DGI patients suggests that this immunologic mechanism may be important in the host's protection against DGI.[20]

The bactericidal activity is also impaired in DGI patients who have complement component deficiencies, particularly terminal complement component deficiencies such as C_5 through C_8.[6] These patients comprise the sole group of patients that may develop recurrent DGI. None of our patients had terminal complement component deficiencies, but one patient was functionally deficient in C_3 activity and another was C_4 deficient. C_3 deficiencies have been associated with recurrent infections caused by encapsulated and Gram-negative organisms.[37] C_4 deficiency may not be associated with an undue susceptibility to infection because the alternative pathway of complement usually is intact.

Since the precise distribution of serum-sensitive and resistant *N. gonorrhoeae* that comprise all strains is not known, the likelihood of any individual becoming colonized with one specific type is also not known. Nevertheless, the majority of strains isolated from patients with complement deficiencies have been serum resistant. The explanation given for increased

Table 6-9
Laboratory Features in Patients with DGI

Patient	Site of isolate	Sensitivity to Normal human serum	Homologous, bactericidal antibody developed
Group I			
1	Blood	0/10	–
2	Blood	0/10	–
3	Pharynx	0/10	–
4	Blood	0/10	–
5	Blood	0/10	–
6	Cervix, rectum	0/10	–
7	Blood, cervix	0/10	–
8	Blood, cervix, rectum	0/10	–
9	Blood	Nd	Nd
10	Pharynx	0/10	+
11	Urethra	0/10	+
12a	Cervix	0/10	–
12b	Cervix	0/10	–
13	Cervix, rectum	Nd	Nd
14	Cervix	0/10	+
15	Blood, cervix	0/10	–
16	Cervix	Nd	Nd
17	Cervix	0/10	+
Group II			
18	Synovial fluid, urethra	3/10	+
19	Synovial fluid, cervix	2/10	+
20	Urethra	2/10	+
21	Cervix	0/10	–
22	Cervix	1/10	+
23	Synovial fluid, cervix	0/10	+
24	Rectum	10/10	+
25	Synovial fluid	0/10	–
26	Synovial fluid	5/10	+
27	Synovial fluid	2/10	+
28	Cervix	8/10	+
29	Urethra	3/10	+
30	Synovial fluid	0/10	–

Nd = Not done

susceptibility to recurrence of DGI in complement deficient patients has been felt to be impaired bacteriolysis. This explanation, however, does not correlate well with the absence of serum-sensitive strains in the complement-deficient patients with DGI. A more likely explanation may be that serum-sensitive strains are usually disposed of locally by polymorphonuclear leukocytes and require only early complement components to stimulate opsonization. In that situation, chemotactic mechanisms usually do not have the opportunity to gain access to the bloodstream, and a bacteriolytic mechanism is not necessary for host defense. In addition, many so-called serum-resistant gonococci may not be serum resistant for all individuals. We have demonstrated this phenomenon in normal individuals, particularly those who have had previous DGI and who have developed bactericidal activity. In those with terminal complement component deficiency, effective bacterolysis, even after previous infection, is never present.

Why do gonococci differ in their sensitivity to the bactericidal system of serum and therefore in their unique capacity to produce specific clinical syndromes? Several mechanisms have been proposed. The laboratory technique utilized to detect serum sensitivity may be important. We tested gonococcal strains against minimally diluted individual normal human sera with use of a low inoculum of organisms to maximize the detection of bactericidal activity.[33] This technique may favor the identification of strains with greater sensitivity that may not be identified using pooled or more diluted serum. Although piliated gonococci have been reported to be more resistant to the lytic action of normal human serum in assays using high inocula,[38] bactericidal susceptibility of gonococci to normal sera was not affected by the state of piliation of organisms in our, and other similarly done, assays.[39,40] We did not, furthermore, observe diminished killing by normal human sera or isogenic, transparent-versus-opaque phenotypes, although transparent phenotypes of highly serum-sensitive strains may be more resistant than their isogenic opaque counterparts.[35] Unique outer membrane protein antigens are present on DGI strains, which may recognize naturally occurring human antibodies. These antibodies, when affixed to gonococci, sterically prevent the binding of bactericidal antibodies directed against lytic target sites.[41] These sites are principally lipopolysaccharide antigens.[42]

Similarly, sera taken from patients early in the course of meningococcal disease may have lytic activity against the infecting strains that is unmasked only when IgA is removed from the sera.[43] Similar inhibition can be demonstrated in the sera of patients who are chronically infected with enteric Gram-negative bacilli and in the IgA fractions of sera taken from patients with brucellosis.[44] The inability of bactericial antibodies to bind to lipopolysaccharide lytic targets may, in turn, prevent effective binding of complement that is needed to complete the lytic attack on the organisms. The membrane attack complex (C 5–9), however, may inadequately insert into the outer membrane of serum-resistant organisms; this thereby precludes the necessary final step in bacteriolysis.

Other unique chemical structures of serum-resistant and sensitive gonococci may also be important in the activation and binding of complement directly or with antibody facilitation. None of the proposed mechanisms that have been offered to explain serum sensitivity or resistance of *N. gonorrhoeae* and their accompanying clinical potential should be considered mutually exclusive. Attempts to explain these mechanisms based solely on the summation of individual effects may fail to take into consideration their possible interrelationships.

THE ROLE OF IMMUNE OR HYPERSENSITIVITY PHENOMENA

The pathogenesis of gonococcal arthritis is usually believed to be due to the direct invasion and replication of *N. gonorrhoeae* in the affected joint. There is, however, significant clinical and laboratory evidence that the arthralgias, tenosynovitis, and dermatitis that are characteristic of DGI may, in part, be due to immune-mediated or hypersensitivity mechanisms (Table 6-10).

Tenosynovitis is the most common musculoskeletal manifestation of DGI. Furthermore, in most patients transient migratory polyarthralgias are the initial symptom and often antedate the onset of tenosynovitis and arthritis. Tenosynovitis and migratory polyarthralgias are common in acute serum sickness and certain infections such as hepatitis, where circulating immune complexes have been incriminated.[45] In contrast, tenosynovitis and migratory polyarthralgias are unusual in nongonococcal bacterial arthritis.[10] The tenosynovitis and migratory polyarthritis are often transient and may completely resolve without antibiotic therapy. Some investigators have postulated that this initial serum sickness-like reaction is related to immune complex phenomena.[46] A transient, aseptic synovitis and/or tenosynovitis may promote the penetration of *N. gonorrhoeae* into affected joints; this results then in a purulent and often culture-positive arthritis.[46]

N. gonorrhoeae can be recovered from less than 50 percent of purulent synovial effusions.[1] This low culture yield is in contrast to nongonococcal bacterial arthritis. Brogidir et al. reported that *N. gonorrhoeae* could be

Table 6-10
Evidence that the Clinical Manifestations of DGI may be due to Aseptic Processes

Predominance of migratory polyarthralgias, dermatitis, and tenosynovitis
Positive synovial fluid culture in less than 50% of purulent effusions
Skin lesions are almost always sterile
Rare positive blood cultures and almost never positive when synovial fluid cultures are positive
Presence of Reiter's syndrome following gonococcal urethritis
Presence of circulating immune complexes
Experimental models of gonococcal arthritis

recovered from only 29 percent of the synovial effusions and in only 3 of 75 blood cultures in their patients with DGI.[9] We found *N. gonorrhoeae* in 47 percent of the synovial effusions and in 26 percent of blood cultures.[1] Of particular interest is the fact that positive blood and positive synovial fluid cultures are not only uncommon but also appear to be mutually exclusive. In thus reviewing a total of 200 patients with DGI recent series, *N. gonorrhoeae* were recovered from 73 synovial effusions and from 50 blood cultures, but only 4 were recovered from both sites (Table 6-5). In contrast, positive blood and synovial fluid cultures occur coincidentally in at least 50 percent of patients with nongonococcal septic arthritis.[10]

The absence of positive cultures from the blood or synovial fluid may be, in part, related to the fastidious growth requirements of *N. gonorrhoeae*.[7,29] Yet *N. gonorrhoeae* can be recovered from the genitourinary tract in most patients with DGI.[1] It is, therefore, possible that the inability to recover *N. gonorrhoeae* from the joint or other site of dissemination can best be explained by immune-mediated or hypersensitivity phenomena. An aseptic synovitis may be initiated or perpetuated by an antigenic component of *N. gonorrhoeae* without the presence of viable organisms. This situation would be analogous to a "reactive" arthritis, such as postulated for Reiter's disease. There are, in fact, similarities of Reiter's disease with gonococcal arthritis since an asymmetrical, acute polyarthritis, urethritis, and dermatitis are common manifestations of both.[11] Scandinavian investigators have reported that aseptic arthritis, indistinguishable from Reiter's syndrome, does follow local gonococcal infections.[28] These reports, however, rely on serologic tests such as the gonococcal complement fixation test, whose diagnostic utility is still controversial.

So called "post infectious" arthritis has also been reported to occur in patients as a manifestation of gonococcal disease.[1] These cases may represent examples of a purulent effusion that persists for days or even weeks, despite sterilization of the synovial fluid by antibiotics. We have treated 2 patients, both of whom developed persistent purulent knee effusions for longer than 10 days after the initiation of appropriate parenteral penicillin therapy. Despite the rapid sterilization of each patient's effusion, large daily synovial fluid effusions continued to accumulate; this required repeated closed-needle aspiration. These effusions contained 20,000–40,000 leukocytes/mm^3. Eventually, the first patient underwent open surgical drainage, joint debridement, and synovectomy. The synovium revealed histologic changes of both acute and chronic synovitis. The second patient received indomethacin 7 days after antibiotics were initiated because of a persistent inflammatory, but sterile, effusion. This persistent effusion largely disappeared a few days after the addition of the anti-inflammatory medication.

The dermatitis associated with DGI also may be due to immune or hypersensitivity mechanisms rather than to septic embolization of *N. gonorrhoeae*. In most large series of DGI, the skin lesions that were cultured have been sterile (Table 6-4). Deposits of immunoglobulin and complement as well as histologic evidence of vasculitis have been reported in these skin lesions.[47] Although the skin lesions are usually described as manculopapular, vesicular, or pustular, erythema nodosum, bullous lesions, and erythema multiforme have been described in patients with DGI.[1] Although *N. gonorrhoeae* are rarely recoverd from these lesions, immunofluorescent staining often reveals evidence of *N. gonorrhoeae*.[29] It has been suggested that a local hypersensitivity phenomena may occur, despite the death of the organisms in the skin. Endotoxin or other inflammatory-provoking stimuli may also be released in these skin lesions.

Serologic evidence for immune phenomena in DGI include the presence of circulating immune complexes. In one report, 13 of 17 patients with DGI had circulating immune complexes detected by either the C1q or the Raji cell assay.[48] In another report, 11 of 12 patients with DGI, compared to only 2 of 12 with local gonococcal infection, had circulating immune complexes detected by the C1q-binding technique.[46] These same authors reported the presence of these complexes early in the synovial fluid and correlated their presence with what was felt to be an initial aseptic synovitis that might promote the later egress of bacteria into the joint. There have also been a few reports of prolonged gonococcal bacteremia that is associated with circulating immune complexes.[49] Finally, as discussed below, experimental models of gonococcal arthritis provide further support for the role of nonviable bacterial components in the pathogenesis of DGI.

LABORATORY MODEL OF DISSEMINATED GONOCOCCAL INFECTION

One of the difficulties in understanding the pathogenesis of DGI relates to the lack of a suitable experimental model.[29] Most investigators have chosen to examine individual aspects of gonococcal disease rather than to study DGI in experimental animals. McGee et al. used human fallopian tube organ cultures to investigate virulence factors.[50] This has been a reliable system to study the virulence potential of various neisserial strains. Type I *N. gonorrhoeae*, a virulent strain, damaged the fallopian tube mucosa more rapidly than type IV, whereas little damage resulted from *N. subflava*.

One of the most important reasons that it has been difficult to develop animal models of gonococcal arthritis relates to the natural antibody levels in experimental animals such as rabbits. Essentially all DGI strains are rabbit serum sensitive, but most are resistant to normal human sera.[29] This normal serum bactericidal activity in laboratory animals makes them resistant to experimental gonococcemia. Recently, investigators have attempted to counter these natural defense mechanisms by implanting devices in the animals to promote prolonged gonococcemia. For example, Arko et al. utilized a subcutaneous chamber device to study urethral infection in chimpanzees.[51] Drutz implanted transaortic valve catheters in rabbits and dogs, and 50 percent of these animals developed gonococcal endocarditis.[52] Although nearly 50 percent of the rabbits developed hepatitis or perihepatitis, none developed arthritis or skin lesions. Twenty percent of the dogs, however, developed arthritis, but multiple injections of *N. gonorrhoeae* were often required. Although these studies were preliminary and often yielded variable results, Drutz did provide evidence that an experimental model of DGI could be devised. The lack of a consistent articular infection may be related to a number of variables that can effect the dissemination of *N. gonorrhoeae* as described above. These include the virulence of the strain of *N. gonorrhoeae*. For example, Drutz found that serum-resistant strains were necessary to cause the experimental endocarditis. Other effectors are the host defense mechansisms. That is, many laboratory animals, such as rabbits, are serum sensitive, e.g., their natural antibody activity is bactericidal to *N. gonorrhoeae*. A third group of effectors include the local defense factors, i.e., the implantation of a chamber or a catheter may provide a "closed space" that prevents normal phagocytosis. In such a closed space, *N. gonorrhoeae* may survive in animals that are "immune" by virtue of their natural antibody activity.

Our own experimental model has employed intra-articular gonococcal injections to take advantage of the closed-space concept.[53] We have developed the first consistently reproducible model of gonococcal arthritis by utilizing intra-articular injections of virulent strains of *N. gonorrhoeae*. *N. gonorrhoeae* isolated from the joint of a patient with gonococcal arthritis and from the blood of a DGI patient caused an acute synovitis followed by a chronic synovitis when injected in rabbits' knees. This particular strain of *N. gonorrhoeae* was resistant to the bactericidal activity of normal human serum, although it was rabbit-serum sensitive. These intra-articular injections of 10^8 *N. gonorrhoeae* caused an acute arthritis within 24 hours after the injection (Fig. 6-1). At 7–10 days, the synovial membrane revealed changes of chronic synovitis with mononuclear leukocyte infiltration as well as deep abscess formation (Fig. 6-2). These changes were histologically identical to those following the injection of 10^8 *Staphylococcus aureus,* hemolytic streptococci, and *Escherichia coli* in rabbits' knees. *N. gonorrhoeae*, however, could not be recovered from the infected joint after 48 hours in any of the rabbits, and most rabbits' joint fluid was sterile 2 hours after the injection. In contrast, the Gram-positive cocci and *E. coli* could be recovered following their injection for days to weeks (Table 6-11).

We then injected killed *N. gonorrhoeae* and lipopolysaccharide isolated and purified from the cell wall of the same strain of *N. gonorrhoeae*. The killed organisms and lipopolysaccharide resulted in a similar acute synovitis followed by a chronic synovitis as described above after the injections of the live organisms.[54] Similar injections of broth and saline controls or of gonococcal outer membrane protein did not cause acute or chronic synovitis.

Table 6-11
Duration of Positive Synovial Fluid Cultures in Rabbits Injected Intra-articularly with *N. gonorrhoeae**

Rabbit	Bacteria injected	Maximum duration of positive synovial fluid cultures (hours)	Day of Sacrifice
1	*N. gonorrhoeae* (blood isolate)	0	1
2	*N. gonorrhoeae* (blood isolate)	0	2
3	*N. gonorrhoeae* (blood isolate)	0	5
4	*N. gonorrhoeae* (blood isolate)	0	7
5	*N. gonorrhoeae* (joint isolate)	2	1
6	*N. gonorrhoeae* (joint isolate)	2	2
7	*N. gonorrhoeae* (joint isolate)	48	7
8	*N. gonorrhoeae* (joint isolate)	2	7
9	*N. gonorrhoeae* (joint isolate)	2	14
10	*N. gonorrhoeae* (joint isolate)	24	28

*In contrast, *Staphylococcus aureus* and group A streptococci could be recovered from the infected joint until the time of sacrifice, and *E. coli* could be recovered for at least 72 hours.

There is thus evidence in this experimental model that nonviable bacterial components will cause an perpetuate an acute and chronic synovitis similar to that following the injection of viable *N. gonorrhoeae*. More research needs to be carried out in such an experimental system to determine the specificity of lipopolysaccharide, as well as the persistence of an antigen–antibody reaction, to document more fully the role of immune and hypersensitivity mechanisms in experimental DGI. Such models of gonococcal arthritis, how-

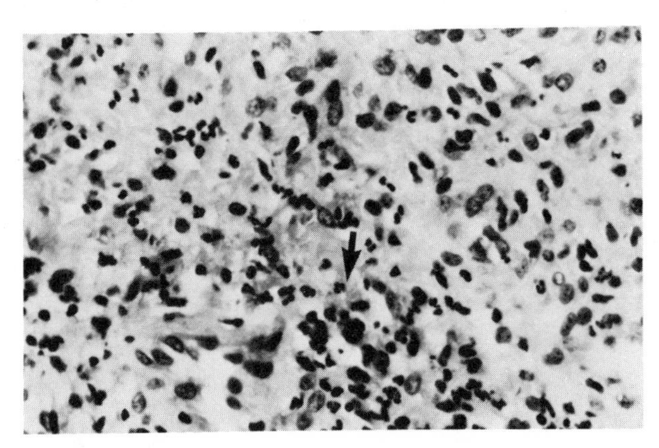

Fig. 6-1. Synovial membrane removed from a rabbit's knee 24 hours after the injection of 10^8 *N. gonorrhoeae* reveals superficial and deep (arrows) infiltration of polymorphonuclear leukocytes. H + E, × 200.

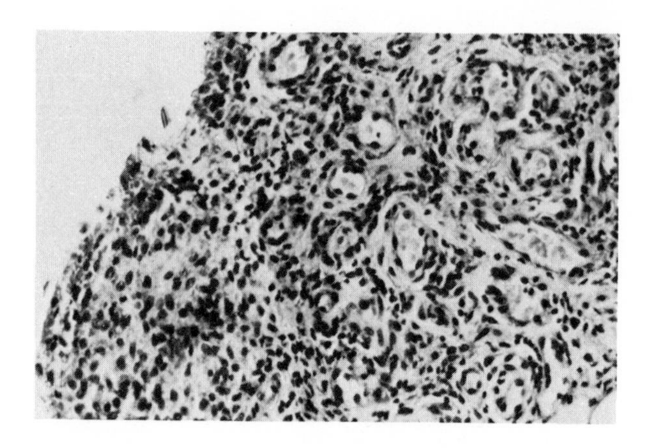

Fig. 6-2. Seven days after the injection of 10^8 *N. gonorrhoeae,* the synovium consists of chronic mononuclear cell infiltrate and granulation tissue. H+E, × 130.

ever, should allow further appreciation of the interactions of the host and the bacteria in this illness.

SUMMARY

DGI is a common illness in most urban medical centers. The clinical manifestations of DGI have changed in the past few decades. DGI now usually occurs in young, healthy females. Tenosynovitis and dermatitis are the most common manifestations. Arthritis may involve a single joint but more often is polyarticular. The genitourinary system will be the best site to recover *N. gonorrhoeae,* whereas the joint, blood, or skin are often sterile. The absence of positive cultures, the serum sickness-like clinical manifestations, and the presence of immunologic evidence of circulating immune complexes point to immune-mediated phenomena in the pathogenesis of features of DGI. Investigators have linked the microbial virulence factors to host resistance features in order to explain why local gonococcal infection disseminates in some patients. These research efforts have, until recently, been hampered by the lack of a suitable experimental model of DGI. Fortunately, the treatment of DGI is still very successful, and almost all patients make a rapid and complete recovery with appropriate antibiotics.

ACKNOWLEDGMENT

This work was supported in part by grants AM-04599, TI-AM 5285, and Multipurpose Arthritis Center Grant AM-20613 from the National Institute of Arthritis, Diabetes, Digestive, and Kidney Diseases, the General Clinical Research Center Grants RR-533 and from the Arthritis Foundation.

REFERENCES

1. O'Brien JP, Goldenberg DL, Rice PA: Disseminated gonococcal infection: A clinical and laboratory survey of 49 patients. Medicine, 62:395–406, 1983
2. Kohen DP: Neonatal gonococcal arthritis: Three cases and review of the literature. Pediatrics 53:436–440, 1974
3. Fink CW: Gonococcal arthritis in children. JAMA 194:237–238, 1965
4. Jacobs NF: Suppurative gonococcal arthritis. JAMA 235:1357, 1976
5. Lee TJ, Utsinger PD, Snyderman R, et al.: Familial deficiency of the seventh component of complement associated with recurrent bacteremic infections due to Neisseria. J Infect Dis 138:359–368, 1978
6. Peterson BH, Lee TJ, Snyderman R, et al.: *Neisseria meningitidies* and *Neisseria gonorrhoeae* bacteremia associated with C_6, C_7, or C_8 deficiency. Ann Intern Med 90:917–920, 1979
7. Holmes KK, Counts GW, Beaty HN: Disseminated gonococcal infection. Ann Intern Med 74:979–993, 1971
8. Chapman DR, Fernandez-Rocha L: Gonococcal arthritis in pregnancy: A ten-year review. South Med J 68:1333–1336, 1975
9. Brogadir SP, Schimmer BM, Myers AR: Spectrum of the gonococcal arthritis–dermatitis syndrome. Semin Arthritis Rheum 8:177–183, 1979
10. Goldenberg DL, Cohen AS: Acute infectious arthritis. Am J Med 60:369–377, 1976
11. Wright V: Arthritis associated with venereal disease: A comparative study of gonococcal arthritis and Reiter's syndrome. Ann Rheum Dis 22:77–90, 1963
12. Metzger AL: Gonococcal arthritis complicating gonorrheal pharyngitis. NEJM 73: 267–269, 1970
13. Cooke DB, Arensberg D, Felner JM, et al.: Gonococcal endocarditis in the antibiotic era. Arch Intern Med 1247–1250, 1979
14. Ebright JR, Komorowski R: Gonococcal endocarditis associated with immune complex glomerulonephritis. Am J Med 68:793–396, 1980
15. Rutkow IM: Gonococcal perihepatitis (the Fitz–Hugh–Curtis syndrome). Am Surg 45:369–373, 1979
16. Keiser H, Ruben FL, Wolinsky E, et al.: Clinical forms of gonococcal arthritis. N Engl J Med 279:234—240, 1968
17. Brandt KD, Cathcart ES, Cohen AS: Gonococcal arthritis: Clinical features correlated with blood, synovial fluid and genito-urinary cultures. Arthritis Rheum 17:502–510, 1974
18. Gelfand SC, Masi AT, Garcia-Kutzbach A: Spectrum of gonococcal arthritis: Evidence for sequential and clinical subgroups. J Rheumatol 2:83–90, 19795
19. Goldman JA: Patterns of gonococcal arthritis. J Rheumatol 8:707–709, 1981
20. Rice PA, Goldenberg DL: Clinical manifestations of disseminated infection caused by *Neisseria gonorrhoeae* are linked to differences in ctericidal reactivity of infecting strains. Ann Intern Med 95:175–178, 1981
21. Garcia-Kutzbach A, Dismuke SE, Masi AT: Gonococcal arthritis: Clinical features and results of penicillin therapy. J Rheumatol 1:210–221, 1974
22. Blankenship RM, Holmes RK, Sanford JP: Treatment of disseminated gonococcal infection. N Engl J Med 290:267–269, 1974
23. Handsfield HH, Wiesner PJ, Holmes KK: Treatment of the gonococcal arthritis–dermatitis syndrome. Ann Intern Med 84:661–667, 1976
24. Trentham DE, McCravey JW, Masi AT: Low-dose penicillin for gonococcal arthritis. JAMA 236:2410–2412, 1976
25. Thompson SE, Rein MF, Jacobs NF, et al.: Gonococcal tenosynovitis-dermatitis and septic arthritis: Intravenous penicillin vs oral erythromycin. JAMA 244:1101–1102, 1980
26. Rinaldi RZ, Harrison WO, Fan PT: Penicillin-resistant gonoccal arthritis. Ann Intern Med 97:43–45, 1982
27. Wiesner PJ, Handsfield HH, Holmes KK: Low-antibiotic resistance of gonococci causing disseminated infection. N Engl J Med 288:1221–1222, 1973
28. Rosenthal L, Olhagen B, Ek S: Aseptic arthritis after gonorrhoeae. Ann Rheum Dis 39:141–146, 1980

29. Eisenstein BI, Masi AT: Disseminated gonococcal infection (DGI) and gonococcal arthritis (GCA): I. Bacteriology, epidemiology, host factors, pathogen factors, and pathology. Sem Arthritis Rheum 10:155–172, 1981
30. Knapp JS, Holmes KK: Disseminated gonococcal infections caused by *Neisseria gonorrhoeae* with unique nutritional requirements. J Infect Dis 132:204–207, 1975
31. Apicella MA, Gaglieardi NC: Antigenic heterogeneity of the non-serogroup antigen of *N. gonorrhoeae*. Infect Immun 26:870–875, 1980
32. Tramont EC, Sadoff JC, Boslego JW, et al.: Gonococcal pilus vaccine. J Clin Invest 68:881–889, 1981
33. Brooks GF, Ingwer I: Studies in the relationships between serum bactericidal activity and uncomplicated genital infections due to *Neisseria gonorrhoeae*. J Infect Dis 138:333–337, 1978
34. Buchanan TM, Hilebrandt JF: Antigen-specific serotyping of *Neisseria gonorrhoeae:* Characterization based upon principal outer membrane protein. Infect Immun 32:985–988, 1981
35. James JF, Swanson J: Color/opacity colonial variants of *Neisseria gonorrhoeae* and their relationship to the menstrual cycle, in Brooks GF, Gotschlilch EC, Holmes KK, Sawyer EB, Young FE (eds): Immunobiology of *Neisseria gonorrhoeae*. Washington, DC, Am Soc Microbiol, 1978
36. Densen P, Markeen LA, Clark RA: Disseminated gonococcal infection is associated with delayed stimulation of complement dependent neutrophil chemotaxis in vitro. Infect Immun 38:563–568, 1982
37. Ballow M, Shira JE, Harden L, et al.: Complete absence of the third component of complement in man. J Clin Invest 56:703–705, 1975
38. McCutchan JA, Levine S, Braude AI: Influence of colony type on susceptibility of gonococci to killing by human serum. J Immunol 116:1652–1655, 1976
39. Tramont EC, Griffiss JM, Rose D, et al.: Clinical correlation of strain differentiation of *Neisseria gonorrhoeae*. J Infect Dis 134:128–131, 1976
40. Tramont EC, Sadoff JC, Artenstein MS: Cross-reactivity of *Neisseria gonorrhoeae* and *Neisseria meningitidis* and the nature of antigens involved in the bactericidal reaction. J Infect Dis 130:240–244, 1974
41. Rice PA, Kasper DL: Characterization of serum resistance of gonococci that disseminate: The role of blocking antibody and outer membrane protein. J Clin Invest 70:157–161, 1982
42. Tramont EC, Sadoff JC, Wilson C: Variability of the lytic susceptibility of *Neisseria gonorrhoeae* to human sera. J Immunol 118:1843–1845, 1977
43. Griffiss JM: Bactericidal activity of meningococcal antisera blocking by IgA of lytic antibody in human convalescent sera. J Immunol 114:1779–1784, 1975
44. Hall WH, Manion RE, Zinneman HH: Blocking serum lysis of *Brucella abortus* by hyperimmune rabbit immunoglobulin A. J Immunol 107:41–46, 1971
45. Duffy J, Lidsky M, Sharp BT: Polyarthritis and hepatitis B. Medicine 55: 19–37, 1976
46. Manicourt DH, Orloff S: Gonococcal arthritis–dermatitis syndrome. Arthritis Rheum 25:574–578, 1982
47. Acherman AB, Miller RCM, Shapiro L: Gonococcemia and its cutaneous manifestations. Arch Dermatol (Chicago) 91:227–232, 1965
48. Walker LC, Ahlin TD, Turg KS, et al.: Circulating immune complexes in disseminated gonorrheal infection. Ann Intern Med 89:28–33, 1978
49. Goldman J, Thompson S III, Jacobs NL: Circulating immune complexes in disseminated gonococcal syndrome. Arthritis Rheum 18:402, 1975
50. McGee ZA, Melly MA, Gregg CR, et al.: Virulence factors of gonococci: Studies using human fallopian tube organ cultures, in Brook GF, Gotschlich EC, Holmes KK, Sawyer WD, Young FE (eds): Immunobiology of *Neisseria gonorrhoeae*. Washington, DC Am Soc Microbiol, 1978
51. Arko RJ, Duncan WP, Brown WJ, et al.: Immunity in infection with *Neisseria gonorrhoeae:* Duration and serologic response in the chimpanzee. J Infect Dis 133:441–447, 1977

52. Drutz D: Hematogenous gonococcal infections in rabbits and dogs, in Brooks, GF, et al (eds): Immunobiology of *Neisseria gonorrhoeae*. Washington, DC, Am Soc Microbiol, 1978
53. Goldenberg DL, Chisholm PL, Rice PA: Experimental models of bacterial arthritis. J Rheumatol 10:1–7, 1983
54. Reed J, Goldenberg DL, Chisholm PL, et al.: Experimental gonococcal arthritis induced by the intra-articular injection of killed bacteria or gonococcal lipopolysaccharide (LPS). Arthritis Rheum 25:S97, 1982

Index